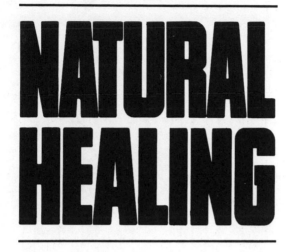

NATURAL HEALING

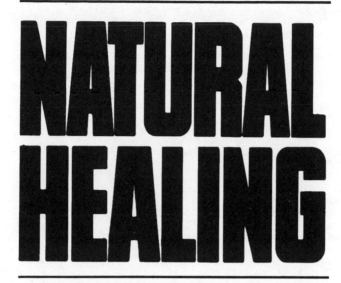

NATURAL HEALING

THE TOTAL HEALTH AND NUTRITION PROGRAM THAT SHOWS YOU HOW TO KEEP YOUR BODY DISEASE-FREE EVERY DAY OF YOUR LIFE

JACK SOLTANOFF, D.C.

WARNER BOOKS

A Warner Communications Company

The author does not directly or indirectly dispense medical advice
or prescribe the use of diet as a form of treatment for sickness
without medical approval. Nutritionists and other experts in the
field of health and nutrition hold widely varying views. It is not
the intent of the author to diagnose or prescribe. The intent is only
to offer health information to help you cooperate with your chosen
health specialist in your mutual quest for health. In the event you
use this information without a health practitioner's approval, you
are prescribing for yourself, which is your constitutional right, but
the publisher and author assume no responsibility.

Printed in the United States of America
First Printing: May 1988
10 9 8 7 6 5 4 3 2 1

Library of Congress Cataloging-in-Publication Data

Soltanoff, Jack.
  Natural healing.

  Includes index.
  1. Naturopathy. I. Title.
RZ440.S64 1988   615.5'35   87-21652
ISBN 0-446-51388-1

Brushing illustrations by Thanh Au
Digestive and other body diagrams by Claudine Heller
Book design by Nick Mazzella

To my gentle, loving wife, Esther,
whose support and encouragement made this book
and so much else possible.
Darling, you will always be in my heart.

Contents

Acknowledgments

My thanks and appreciation to my children, my colleagues, Dr. Ruth Soltanoff and Dr. Howard Soltanoff, for their indispensable help and assistance. Jerry Celente and Mary Ann Celente of the Socio-Economic Research Institute of America are due particular thanks for their encouragement in initiating this project. I have drawn unhesitatingly from the extensive files of the Institute for the research data that provides this book with its factual base. Thanks to my thousands of supportive patients, especially those whose testimonials bear witness to the efficacy of Natural Healing, I owe a profound debt. Thanks to the authors of the thousands of books whose wisdom I have culled and to the courageous and far-sighted founders of chiropractic who have made my own practice so rewarding. Thanks to John Anthony West for responding to a literary S.O.S.; and thanks to Claire Peters, Leslie Keenan of Warner Books, Sue Nirenberg, Gary Abatelli, Ron Villane, John Melia, Roberta Sickler, Dr. Louis Sportelli, the American Chiropractic Association and the many others who in their various capacities made the writing of this book the extraordinary experience it was.

Foreword

How can I be responsible for my health? My child's always getting sick; what can I do to change that? What about the environment? What impact does that have on my health? On my children's health? Use this book to answer some of these questions. It provides an opening, a space for you to see what you can do about your health and what's standing in your way.

This book is an exciting book, an important book. One that focuses on the basics of what goes into your body and what happens to it: intake and elimination.

As I was sitting down to write this, I read an article in a recent Sierra magazine entitled 'No safe harbor for marine life.' This was about a chemical called TBT that the Navy wants to use to paint the hulls of boats. This might be the most toxic substance we could deliberately place in the environment (as bad as DDT), and it would remain active in the environment indefinitely. Our lives are under constant attack—directly and indirectly. Pesticides, food additives, microwaves, radiation, high voltage wires—all of these bombard our defenses: our immune system, liver (the detoxifier in our body), adrenal glands. Our bodies have to work overtime to do what they were designed to do naturally. In my practice as a medical doctor, I see the results: hyperactivity, allergies, recurrent ear infections, immune problems (AIDS and Epstein Barr among them), PMS. The list goes on. To treat these we need a holistic approach, one that integrates mind, body, and spirit.

In other words, if our bodies are getting bombarded with too many substances, if we're not putting in the right substances and amounts, if we're not eliminating properly, if our body is not distributing and balancing the products of digestion both biochemically and energetically, then disease results. In treating a disease process we have to think about all these parameters and either change them or reverse them in order to effect a cure. In prevention, we have to take into account our own personal genetic strengths and weaknesses and not fall victim to them. This is exactly what Dr. Soltanoff's book is about. He shows you ways to help yourself get healthy if you're sick and ways to help yourself stay healthy if you already are.

As a physician, I see Dr. Soltanoff's combination of nutrition, exercise, and dry brushing as a sound and original concept. His dry brushing (a form of skin massage) is based upon Acupuncture principles. If you're stimulating your skin, you're stimulating your whole body. Acupuncture theory deals with the body as an electroenergetic unit, one in which different kinds of energy (food, air, spiritual) are taken in, assimilated, and distributed to continually recharge the body and all its parts in a cyclic fashion—on a daily, hourly, seasonal basis. The body is like a hologram. The whole body is represented by each of its parts. That is to say, the surface of the body reflects what is happening inside—to the liver, the stomach, the kidneys, etc.

If we as individuals can understand the workings of restructuring our health from a responsible place (ourselves), then we can go forth and make a difference to others and society in general, which will eventually make a better environment in the world and so will come back to us and nurture us. I see Dr. Soltanoff's program as a strong foundation, something to build on.

Steven Bock, M.D.
Board Certified Family Practice
New York State Certified in Acupuncture
Co-Director: Rhinebeck Health Center
                    Rhinebeck, N.Y. 12572

Introduction

In this book, I will show you how to prevent disease, how to rejuvenate your body, and how to enjoy a healthy, active long life. Every cell, every tissue, every organ, every system in your body can be revitalized through the step-by-step plan I call Biochemical Reprogramming. I will explain how the unbeatable triple combination of nutrition, exercise, and my unique acupuncture-based skin brushing technique invigorates and activates your nervous system, your digestive system, and your endocrine (glandular) system. When these three systems function optimally—and they should if you follow my program—your health swiftly improves and stays improved.

You Are Responsible for Your Own Health

In the final analysis, *you* are the person primarily responsible for improving and then maintaining your health on a long-term basis—with some direction, of course. Over many decades of clinical experience, I have seen thousands of supposedly incurable, chronically ill patients show remarkable improvement, even after years of downhill health—many recovering to the point where they are in better health than ever before. And they keep improving, doing things each year that they were unable to do for years, gradually developing more strength, more energy, and more endurance, and appreciating their newfound health every moment of each day. What was responsible for their ill health? For the most part, unbalanced, commercialized, almost valueless diets combined with sedentary living and lack of exercise are bound to lead to acute and/or chronic disease.

Nutrition Is the
Key to Health

Your body is a mirror of what you eat, drink, and think daily. There can be no doubt about this. What does it take to sustain your health and build your body every day of your life? Certainly not drugs. Certainly not contaminants such as caffeine. Certainly not toxins such as sugar. Certainly not devitalized white flour. The correct foods necessary to maintain your health, energy, and well-being are of paramount importance and must be eaten daily. Once you learn to apply the basics of this nutrition program, better health automatically follows. Some of the foremost experimental medical laboratories have been able to produce various acute and chronic diseases at will through nutritional controls. Their research has revealed that the absence, deficiency, or imbalance of one or more nutritional factors such as vitamins, minerals, enzymes, and unsaturated fats produced various states of acute or chronic disease. A return to a balanced, nutritious diet eliminated these health problems very quickly.

Our Appetites No Longer Enslave Us;
Old Age No Longer Frightens Us

The importance of nutrition to health is not a new discovery. Nutrition has had its passionate advocates for decades, but their advice usually went unheeded. But today there is abundant proof that these early crusaders for the natural approach—and I include myself!— were right, and their sneering, well-publicized critics wrong. Many informed people now recognize that the basic insights propounded by these early pioneers have been substantiated by contemporary research. Social awareness, particularly among younger people, has advanced our society to the point where health food stores and fitness centers flourish in just about every town and city in this country. They are integrating this important information into their lifestyles to survive in this stressful, polluted age.

From my perspective, a perspective based on decades of clinical practice, in every consideration of health and disease, correct nutrition ranks number one. So this book focuses primarily on how your food is broken down and assimilated. I will discuss the relationship of food and nutrition to your future health and happiness, well-being, and longevity.

Physiological, psychological, and sociological factors can affect one's health and happiness. However, with correct nutrition, exercise, daily skin brushing, and moderation in every area of your life, good health should naturally follow. The aging process should automatically slow down, resulting in longer life, a life free from crutches, walkers, wheelchairs, and the indignity of nursing homes. A life in which you have the independence and mobility to take care of yourself.

Personal Priorities

Correct nutrition is a question of personal priorities; it is not a starvation diet or a so-called fad diet. What do you consider more important: overeating and digestive ailments, smoking and lung cancer, drinking and liver disease, sedentary living and obesity, *or* physical well-being, mental clarity, sexual vigor, and graceful aging with minimally impaired vision and hearing? Laboratory studies show that simple but balanced nutritious meals tend to decrease the incidence of and/or to postpone many serious diseases, including obesity, diabetes, arteriosclerosis (hardening of the arteries), coronary disease, and cancer.

I have dedicated my entire life to the concept that everyone should become more concerned with the quality of his or her life. To that end, I have written this book, which is literally a love offering. It's a long-term dream come true—a means of sharing my successes with you and offering you health alternatives outside the mainstream. If we all live healthier and think healthier, we can link together to help solve the ecological, social, and political problems of our planet. We should all share a common goal for a happier, healthier, more positive future.

CHAPTER 1

My Philosophy, My Practice, My Intentions

Although the average medical doctor spends less than five minutes with each patient to explain the nature of an ailment, I put no limit on the time I spend with each nutritional patient. My colleagues think I am crazy to spend so much time with my patients; but *physician* means "teacher" and "educator" in Greek, and that's what I do with each and every patient—*teach and educate*. Unfortunately, most medical doctors do not focus on teaching and educating. They are primarily interested in relieving the symptoms, not finding the cause. I know this from my patients who come to me after seeing the top specialists in different fields. (I call myself the Last-Resort Doctor.) And what I want to do in this book is teach you—teach you how your own body works and how you (and only you) can make yourself completely healthy.

Whereas the typical doctor prescribes medication, I give my patients a prescription for living. Numerous studies conducted by the federal government, the National Research Council's Committee on Medical Education, and the National Academy of Sciences reveal that medical schools fail to emphasize nutrition. One report specifically states that despite growing evidence of the importance of diet in disease prevention, United States medical schools cram future doctors full of technical know-how and teach too little about food and nutrition. In contrast, I have spent many years studying and applying the benefits of proper nutrition. Over the years I've developed a unique system I call Biochemical Reprogramming. In this book you'll learn what this system is and how to use it to heal yourself and stay healthy. But first let me explain how I, a chiropractor, became involved in nutrition and healing. I was, of course, brought up in a vastly different world from the world we live in today.

When Food Was Food

When I was a boy in the early 1900s—ah, how foods tasted then! When you bit into a tomato, you knew you were eating a tomato! Of course, you only ate tomatoes in season. Today you eat tomatoes in January. They may look red and appealing, but they are tasteless and tough. They've been tampered with chemically and genetically. They have little nutrient value.

As if to compensate for the tastelessness of such intensively grown produce, the rest of our food has been artificially jazzed up. We live in a world of perverted cravings. When you take in the proper nutrients at a meal, you don't have those cravings for sweets later on. If your body is satisfied, as it is when you eat correctly, your taste buds quickly normalize. Today in America people literally pervert their own taste buds; a whole chain reaction takes place. Once you start with sugary foods, for instance, you just want more and more because a chemical imbalance is created. Once you have freed yourself from sugar, your natural instincts can come to the fore and your perverted cravings will gradually disappear.

Then and Now

In my day those who were aware of the connection between food and health were called "health nuts" and "cranks." Health foods and the health food industry have come a long way from the era of so-called eccentricity, the heyday of Bernarr MacFadden, William Howard Hays, Adolph Just, Louis Kuehne, Father Kniepp, Benedict Lust, and George Bernard Shaw. I confess that as a young boy (when this story begins), I had not heard of them. I was thinking about my childhood hero, Benjamin Franklin, who wrote:

Dine with little, sup with less:
Do better still; sleep supperless.
Be not sick too late, nor well too soon.
An ounce of prevention is
worth a pound of cure.
How much easier it is to keep well
than to get well.

Benjamin Franklin has been my role model from my earliest days. As the son of Russian immigrant parents, growing up in Newark, New Jersey and eager to make my mark in the world, I was more impressed with the accomplishments of Ben Franklin than with those of any other patriot. He was eighty-four years old when he died, and few persons, before or since, have achieved so much in so many different endeavors. Franklin did the work of six men, and did it uncommonly well.

How was it possible for one man with none too strong a constitution to perform so much in so many fields—science, invention, literature, education, politics, and business? Again and again in his writings, Franklin revealed his secret: "From earliest manhood," he wrote, "I was resolved to make the guarding of my health a first consideration." Indeed, throughout his long life Franklin never neglected an ailment, never permitted a malady, no matter how trifling, to go unattended. His whole philosophy of health is summed up in his admonition, "When you are well, keep well." I know knowledgable readers may ask about Ben's undeniable belly, and how about all the women and all the wine? It's true, but Franklin seems to have mastered the art of excess in moderation. He knew when to stop. And in fact there's something of that understanding built into Biochemical Reprogramming with its two "eat what you want" days.

Few men in any era have been so thoroughly alive, physically and mentally, as Franklin. But without the glowing health to which he attended so assiduously, his remarkable record would have been impossible. Had he neglected his treasured asset, the name of Franklin would not have been held in esteem for centuries.

A Fortunate Accident

Believing pharmacology was the key to the health that Franklin so admired, I planned to become a pharmacist. In the 1920s when I was a teenager, I worked six and a half days a week as a drugstore delivery boy at a salary of two dollars a week. One day while I was delivering a prescription, a hit-and-run driver knocked me off my bike. I was in excruciating pain, but with the vigor of a thirteen-year-old, I was able to stagger several miles to my house. When I went to the bathroom, I saw a sight that frightened me more than the pain: blood in my urine. My parents, who were both home at the time, called the doctor, and I was taken off on a stretcher to the hospital. The doctors told my parents I had fractured my spine and ribs and ruptured my kidneys. They planned to remove my left kidney, but I wouldn't let them operate. (Even as a boy I had an intuitive feeling about invasive procedures.)

Since the doctors weren't sure how to relieve the pain or stop the bleeding of a nonconforming, uncooperative patient, they were helpless. Finally they told my parents to accept the fact that their son would be gone in a year. Gone in a year! Their only son! Luckily a distant relative gave my parents the name of a chiropractor (what was *that*?). Initially he prescribed a healing nutrition program, a procedure that was unheard of at the time. After the fractures healed, he gradually and gently straightened out my twisted body frame through chiropractic adjustment. He gave Tuesday night lectures on nutrition at a Newark club called the Bona Vita ("good life" in Latin). At the Bona Vita (where I met my future wife Esther), this chiropractor took his place in my life alongside Benjamin Franklin as a role model, and turned my thinking around. I put away boyhood fancies: the idea of becoming a pharmacist, my sister's chocolate icing, my mother's homemade cakes, and herring.

After I started hanging out at the Bona Vita, I redefined my lifestyle, literally walking miles to buy day-old whole wheat bread and whole wheat muffins at Dugan's Bakery. My parents were rigid in their ways, but they encouraged my new eating style even though they rejected it personally. That was a tragic mistake. My father, a cigar lover and heavy beef eater, died of stomach cancer at the age of forty-eight. And my mother, who despite hypertension ate salted herring for breakfast every morning, suffered three strokes and died six weeks later, also at forty-eight.

How's that for a genetic background! Although a genetic weakness may undermine our health somewhat, I tell my patients not to use their genetic heritage as an excuse to go on filling their bellies with poison. A change to healthier eating and living habits from those of our parents and grandparents will help us avoid the diseases that plagued them. When people tell me my robust health and longevity must be due to genetics, I point out the early deaths of my parents.

Okay, I was not totally perfect. In my late teens I wanted to look sophisticated, so despite my new ways of eating, I took up cigarette smoking. I knew that nicotine constricted the arteries and filled the lungs with tar, but I didn't know about the addictive substances and additives in cigarettes. (After I started practicing chiropractic, I didn't want my patients to see me huffing and puffing on a cigarette, so I gave up the weed.) People worry about wrinkled skin, not realizing that smoking creates a murky invisible internal wrinkling as well. After all, cigarettes are another chemical you ingest. I felt rotten when I smoked. When I realized I didn't need artificial stimulation (or the look of sophistication), I became dedicated to the pursuit of health, an "eccentric" maybe, but not entirely alone in my convictions.

I was recently reminded of my youthful self-righteousness when I read in *The New York Times* about a show at the Hudson River Museum in Yonkers called "Fit for America: Health, Fitness, Sport and American Society, 1830 to 1940":

> "We of the last quarter of the twentieth century did not invent health foods, aerobics or exercise machines," said Dr. Harvey Green, curator of a new museum show that explores the history of the great American urge to shape up, eat right and stay well. "Back then, staying in shape was not only a personal quest," Dr. Green said, "but a spiritual imperative."

What Is Chiropractic?

As a young follower of those whose spiritual imperatives demanded "shaping up, eating right, and staying well," I traded in my plan to become a pharmacist for a better one. Following in the footsteps of the man who had literally saved my life, I would become a chiropractor. Chiropractic is a health discipline. It is based upon the premise that the relationship between structure and function in the human body is a significant health factor and that relationships between the spinal column and the nervous system contribute to the disease process. Simply put, chiropractic is concerned mainly with the spine. Nerves radiating from the spine supply your entire body with life and energy, and your health depends upon the unimpeded flow of this nervous energy. When pressure upon nerves interferes with or slackens the energy flow, you feel ill or fatigued; you may or may not feel pain. In other words, you know something is wrong, but you may not realize the spine is involved. Unless this condition is corrected, illness may result. The primary objective of chiropractic is to relieve nerve pressure by balancing and integrating the skeletal framework. In a chiropractic adjustment, the chiropractor releases nerve pressure by gently readjusting the spine manually, thus opening the channels of healing and repair. Taking painkillers or other drugs blocks the nervous system and can adversely affect the immune system as well as the digestive system. If you take painkillers and undergo chiropractic adjustments at the same time, you work against yourself. It's like driving a car with one foot on the gas and one on the brake. In short, these symptom-relieving drugs are to all intents and purposes useless and potentially dangerous.

While studying at Mecca College of Chiropractic in Newark, I learned in detail about Daniel David Palmer, originally a grocer and teacher who became a healer and eventually "the father of chiropractic." It seems that in September 1890, a janitor named Harvey Lillard, who was so deaf that he could not hear the rumbling of wagons in the street, learned of Palmer's healing expertise and entered his office for help. Lillard explained that seventeen years earlier, while lifting something heavy in a cramped, stooped position, he had felt something snap in his back and had been deaf ever since. On examining Lillard, Palmer located a prominent displaced vertebra in the neck. Palmer knew that the acoustic nerve was connected to this vertebra. He reasoned that if the vertebra were repositioned, Lillard's hearing might be restored. Palmer then applied a short thrust with his hand, which realigned the vertebra, which in turn released the impinged nerve. Soon afterward Lillard's hearing returned to normal. Chiropractic was born! Inspired by

Palmer (as well as Ben Franklin) and imbued with chiropractic zeal, which I've maintained through the years, I began to practice.

In those days it was illegal to practice chiropractic, but I chose it as a profession because I believed in it right down to the tips of my toes. Finally in the fifties, because of grass-roots pressure from patients who wrote letters to their legislators, the states began to issue licenses. Today chiropractors are licensed in every state in the union. But before we were accepted as totally legitimate, I had been handcuffed, fingerprinted, and sentenced for the "crime" of practicing drugless medicine: chiropractic and natural healing. (After being bailed out of jail by my wife, I invariably ended up with suspended sentences.)

I continued to read on my own and take courses everywhere, from Iceland to Greece to Yugoslavia. With a kernel of truth here, a kernel of truth there, four years of night school at the accredited Chiropractic Institute of New York to become licensed, plus my experience over the years, I gradually put it all together.

Living a Healthy Life
Wasn't Easy When I Started Out

I could count on the ridicule of my smoking and drinking friends and relatives when they visited us. My cousin, a dentist who taught dentistry at the University of Pennsylvania and at Seton Hall in New Jersey, used to call me an oddball. Despite his taunts, we entrusted our teeth and our children's teeth to him. However, to his bewilderment, he was never able to find any cavities in our children's teeth. I said, "Doesn't this prove conclusively that the regime we live under and what we do is correct?"

Looking me straight in the eye, he said, "It's purely an accident of birth," and turned around and slammed the door. This attitude is typical of many health professionals who "slam the door" on the mounting evidence supporting natural healing. And for the record, my cousin's son became a chiropractor.

Bringing Up Children

People ask me if Esther and I brought up our children, two daughters and a son, according to the precepts of health that we learned at the Bona Vita. We did. At first we gave them Walker-Gordon certified raw milk (no longer available), which was delivered to our house, and fruits and vegetables. Certainly people were unaware (as many still are) that modified diet and correct eating are the way to avoid disease. We didn't force anything with our children. We never made our way of life a prison sentence. We never dragged them kicking and screaming to the table or threatened them with doom if they ate cakes and cookies at a friend's house. We simply set a good example. Our neighbors weren't interested in healthful breads and vegetables, so my children, with their sandwiches of whole wheat bread in a white-bread era, were often the butts of jokes and ridicule by the other children. Their breakfasts were basically the same as those of most children—and yet they were different. We gave them millet, an alkaline protein cereal, and fresh fruit. For school lunch, they would take along a lettuce, tomato, and cucumber sandwich, carrot or celery sticks, or a sandwich made of freshly ground nut butter, and an apple or pear. For supper, we all ate primarily vegetarian—and we ate very well indeed. (See chapter 6.) At birthday parties, they enjoyed ice cream and cake.

They never rebelled, and there were no problems with any of them. They saw that neither of us drank or served alcohol or smoked. They saw that our neighbors were susceptible to a variety of illnesses and we weren't. The kids had a bit of a hard time, but as they grew older we just left reading material around on health. Instead of cake, candy, and ice cream, Esther would leave little dishes of sunflower and pumpkin seeds or raisins and currants around the house. (Yes, it is possible to bring up children *happily* on a healthful diet. See "School Lunches for Kids," pages 117-18.) The final result? Two of our three children grew up to become chiropractors and proponents of the natural healing lifestyle, and our third child, now a judge, follows it partially. And since they rarely saw their parents tired or sick (Esther died several years ago of complications resulting from an automobile accident involving a drunken driver), it is not surprising that our children followed in our footsteps. My college-student granddaughter Naomi, a third-generation follower, says, "Grandpa, I'm the only one at college who never catches a cold."

How My Practice Developed and
What It Is Today

In the mid-1950s, Esther and I decided to leave Newark. I had always liked Greenwich Village in New York City, and I felt that Village people would be advanced in their thinking. New York was the place to go! My lawyer and accountant were opposed to this move, but Esther and I were for it. Space was at a premium, but I was able to rent and renovate a little candy store across from a Franciscan church.

Until I got my Village practice going, I tapered off my New Jersey practice. I would see my last patient in Newark at four or five o'clock and drive to New York, an hour away. Then I'd work in my New York office straight through midnight. I managed this schedule for a couple of years and eventually converted a former Beech-Nut warehouse on west Houston Street to an office with seven adjustment rooms. By that time nutritional counseling had become an integral part of my chiropractic practice, and as my practice started to mushroom, I took on an associate, then another and another, winding up with three full-time and three part-time chiropractors, but I still spent time with and monitored the progress of each patient.

When I first started my practice, I very rarely saw heart attack patients under the age of sixty-five. Today I see men and women who have had massive coronaries in their thirties and even their twenties. By the time they're in their thirties today, many men and women have developed one or more chronic health problems, some of which are potentially crippling or fatal. Statistics may show increased longevity, but in my opinion this is due to sophisticated technology and improved sanitation. Overall health is worse.

Live Longer—but Live Sicker?

Another factor responsible for increased longevity, in my opinion, is the unions. You no longer see women working twelve to sixteen hours a day in sweatshops with unguarded machinery, filthy bathrooms, and windows that won't open in the summertime and won't close in the wintertime, as was the norm when my mother worked.

Unions have dramatically changed working conditions. Because of this, people do live longer, but the average older person lives with a host of debilitating ailments; number one among these, and the chief cause of death in America, is cardiac disease. (During the Korean War, the U.S. Army Medical Corps autopsied 2,000 American boys between the ages of eighteen and twenty-three, the flower of American manhood. They found that 84 percent had already developed atherosclerosis, narrowing of the arteries, and arteriosclerosis, hardening of the arteries around the heart, and were candidates for heart attack by the ages of forty, forty-five, or fifty. If this is true of boys between eighteen and twenty-three, you can just picture the health of the average mature American.)

When I started practicing as a chiropractor, we mostly treated patients who had problems of neuro-muscular-skeletal origin. Occasionally other open-minded people whose ailments would not respond to orthodox treatment would try chiropractic. Many responded to spinal manipulation, but if not, I would seek alternatives. I noticed as time went on that more and more people were not responding as quickly as others had in the past. What was the matter? I began to realize that their sluggish response was due to a poor level of general health, that the response to spinal manipulation was better when I first started out because general health was better. Thus, I developed a nutritional program with receptive patients, and through proper diet, these patients revitalized their bodies and became more resilient and more responsive to chiropractic adjustments.

Greener Pastures

Nineteen years ago we left the congestion and increasing pollution of city living for greener pastures. We took up roots in the Woodstock, New York area—a rural artistic colony nestled in the foothills of the Catskill Mountains. I believed I would have little difficulty establishing myself in this cultural community that seemed like an extension of Greenwich Village. The beauty and tranquillity of Woodstock makes it an ideal community in which to retire. Actually I've tried to retire three times. Retirement might work for others, but it does not work for me. When I read what the composer Jule Styne, then eighty-one years old, said about retirement, it struck a responsive chord: "I'm working harder, thinking better, being able to listen to other people better—that comes from getting older. I never stop to think about my age. The whole name of the game is, you must have something to do every day, so you just can't wait till you do it. You've got to go to a place where you sit down and do some work. Your brain *wants* to work. It worked all your life for you. If you want to retire, you're old. If you keep your brain working, you're young."

My typical day begins with fifteen minutes of calisthenics. I see my first patient at eight in the morning and continue to work until I break for a short nap around three in the afternoon. I follow the nap with a regular exercise program including a range of activities from walking to weight training. I continue working and keep going until midnight or one. As a rule, I eat only one meal a day —dinner. I believe that's why I'm going strong long past Social Security age! When I was younger I would eat two apples or a few pears and a handful of nuts in the middle of the day. I found out purely by accident that if I skipped lunch because I was too busy to eat, I felt better. Later on in the evening I'll eat fruit. I like simplicity and I like to eat the same thing each day. I have never ever counted a single calorie, and you won't have to either. This doesn't mean that my strict regime is the right one for you, but when you're on a program of natural healing, you count productive years—not calories or carbohydrates.

The Importance of Daily Rest

Besides good nutrition and moderate exercise, the secret of my energy is a daily forty-five-minute rest. You don't have to sleep, but you should lie absolutely horizontal or on a slantboard (see p. 261) to take the pressure off your heart, lungs, liver, kidneys, and brain. You equalize your body fluids, giving your body a chance to revitalize itself.

I Practice What I Preach

I'm not a hypocrite with a big potbelly, a cigarette in his fingers, and a hearing aid, who says, "Do as I say, not as I do." I believe a health doctor must set a living example to his patients. For more than fifty years I have lived the program I share with you in this book. I won't suggest a diet that you must eat like a horse with blinders. Once a week or so, I go to a Chinese restaurant (though I ask that no MSG be added to my food) or eat ice cream, which I dearly love. So you sin *occasionally*, so what! When I get home, I drink a glass of warm water and fresh squeezed lemon juice to neutralize it. Frequently patients ask if they can go off the program on special occasions: a slice of birthday cake at a friend's party, for example. I say, "Of course. We only pass this way once."

My practice keeps me going. I'll tell you, I'm on cloud nine all the time because I see improvements—*dramatic* improvements—in my patients as they switch from high-powered, potentially dangerous medication to a simpler nutritional program. Unfortunately, I don't think the average orthodox doctor sees such remarkable improvements or experiences this kind of fulfillment.

My 600-Question Questionnaires vs. Medical Testing

Do you "go to pieces" easily, dislike working under pressure? Is your behavior erratic, "flighty"? Do you have an unaccountable burning on the soles of your feet? Do you sigh and yawn frequently? These are just four out of six hundred questions I would ask you on questionnaires I gradually compiled, which focus on different health problems. When you come in as a patient seeking nutritional counseling, I give you these questionnaires to complete at home. The questions are designed to identify health problems in specific systems and organs. Redundancies and a system of checks and cross-checks are integrated into the questionnaires in order to ensure their accuracy and reliability. My questionnaires detect not only existing health problems but incipient ones as well. The accurate diagnosis and the subsequent recovery of innumerable patients has led me to believe my questionnaires are much more comprehensive and valid than many medical tests. Once I determine what the problems are, I explain exactly what is happening in your body, where it happens, and what Biochemical Reprogramming must take place in order to arrest the condition. At this point I am prepared to design a tailor-made nutritional program for each patient. The more questions the patient asks, the happier I am, because this is how the patient becomes more knowledgeable and deeply committed to the program.

How Does a Chiropractor/Nutritionist
Detect a Health Problem?

In addition to the questionnaires, I employ a unique variety of diagnostic techniques. As a holistic practitioner trained in integrating all the systems of the body, I have learned to recognize subtle clues frequently ignored by typical orthodox practitioners.

I can tell a lot by just noticing what *you* might call surface— even cosmetic—details. I note the state of your hair, for example. Is it brittle? Is it oily? Is it dry? Is it resilient? I note the whites of your eyes. Are they cloudy? Are they bloodshot, lined with tiny or thickened veins? I note your skin. Is it pasty or pale? Do you have blackheads? Acne? I note your nails. I look at the ridges, to see if they reveal a deficiency of calcium or protein. I note your speech, and I note whether your movements are jerky. I note your posture and whether you lean forward to hear when I speak. All these signs are barometers of your health. I even note a part of you that you are barely aware of: your tongue. Yes, it is true, even your tongue tells a doctor more about your state of health than you ever dreamed possible. It can tell him or her not only about your present state of health but about what happened to you years ago. For example, a fifty-eight-year-old executive who recently went to a new doctor for a checkup had not even disrobed for examination when the doctor inquired, "How long ago did you have a stroke?"

"Stroke?" echoed the patient. "Yes, I did have a mild one twelve years ago. How in the world could you tell?"

The doctor explained, "As you were speaking to me, I noticed that your tongue moved to one side instead of straight ahead. This inability of the tongue to protrude in the midline is often the aftermath of a stroke."

The direction in which the tongue moves is one clue your doctor can use to determine the location and extent of different types of nerve damage. To understand this, we must remember that until shortly before we are born, we have not one tongue but two. Before birth the tongue exists in the mouth as two separate sections, a right and a left half.

These two halves then fuse together, as indicated by the furrow extending down the middle of the tongue. Since each half of the tongue has its own nerve supply, the normal movements of the tongue are the result of a delicate balance between the right and left hemispheres of the brain. Therefore, in order for a normal person to be able to thrust his tongue straight ahead, a perfect balance must exist between the nerves of the right and left halves of the tongue. If a right nerve is damaged or paralyzed, the muscles in the right half will fail to act, so that the muscles on the left will thrust the tongue forcibly outward to the right. As a result the tongue will behave like a car with its right wheel suddenly braked—it will veer to the right. Such a reaction is usually due to cerebral hemorrhage (stroke), shock, or trauma.

Twenty-four centuries ago, Hippocrates knew that a coated or furred tongue reflected conditions from colds and fevers to liver, gallbladder, digestive, and kidney disorders. However, recent medical studies show other causes. In Turin, Italy, Dr. Beno Dorn, in a study of seven hundred patients, found that many people with coated tongues were moderate or heavy smokers. He also found that constantly furred tongues were associated with diseases of the respiratory tract. About 30 percent had an infection of ear, nose, or throat. His findings also showed that sore throat or tonsillitis was a common cause of a coated tongue, but that tooth decay, no matter how bad, could not be the cause. The latest research is now transforming the tongue into a major diagnostic tool.

Many people who come to see me for the first time tell me how healthy they are: "I just want an evaluation." Filling out my questionnaires makes them very much aware that they aren't as healthy as they thought they were and that potentially serious health problems are brewing internally. They become aware that prevention beats drugs and surgery.

I frequently change a patient's entire lifestyle through gradual steps, not just nutritionally, but through exercise, fresh air, rest, sleep, sunshine, and relief of stress. Each phase of life is planned out for each patient on an individual basis. So instead of superficial painkilling or symptom-masking drugs, a patient receives a positive health improvement plan for life, with periodic reevaluations. Patients receive these same questionnaires every four to six weeks as a basis for comparison, and as they feel better and their symptoms subside, I gradually modify their programs so they are easily integrated into their daily routines.

Does a new patient accept this method immediately? Some do, some don't. Often a patient will say, "Dr. Soltanoff, how do you know what is wrong with me without an X-ray?" My answer is this: "I have been practicing for years and years, and your case is familiar. Through these comprehensive questionnaires and my evaluation of you, I usually recognize the problem." If I suspect a malignancy (or similar catastrophic illness), I will refer you to an appropriate, competent medical practitioner.

In my rather large practice, I rarely X-ray more than four or five people in one year. Why not? Because not much in your body ever happens overnight. For example, an EKG tells you what is happening at that moment only; it does not comprehensively detect all potential cardiac maladies. There are many different heart problems, and the EKG detects some but not all. What is the value of a nonconclusive EKG? A familiar scenario is "John Doe went for an EKG, got a clean bill of health, walked out the door, and had a heart attack."

If you find my views on medical testing offbeat, you may be surprised to learn that both the American College of Physicians and the nation's largest insurer, Blue Cross/Blue Shield, say that *about 20 percent of all diagnostic tests are unwarranted*, and they have developed guidelines to determine when fifteen commonly performed medical tests are unnecessary.

A New Human Science

I've refined my techniques over the years to practice what I call Biochemical Reprogramming, which goes far beyond "curing" disease in the conventional manner. It is a marriage of metabolic nutrition, exercise, skin brushing, biochemistry, drugless medicine, dynamic breathing techniques, and some herbal and food supplements. It detects and alerts the patient to bodily predisease changes. In my practice today I look for the deep underlying causes of discomfort or disease. Then I set up an individual program to reeducate the patient's mind and body. I change taste buds and appetite as well as eating, exercise, and breathing habits. In my practice I give the patient direction, support, and new hope. This is what I hope to do for you in the chapters ahead. I hope to teach you to recognize and correct your own health problems, to avoid future ills, and to achieve a happier, healthier, more efficient, and pain-free life.

As our bodies struggle to stay well and vigorous to an advanced age, we must individually accept the responsibility for our own health and, avoiding drugs and surgery whenever possible, work patiently and conscientiously toward that end. Step by step, day by day, as you embrace each element of this program, you will feel yourself revitalized as you progress on the path toward natural healing.

CHAPTER 2

Biochemical Reprogramming: How to Fight the Conspiracy Against Your Health

We know that the causes of disease are legion. As a chiropractor, I regard spinal misalignments as a factor most immediately related to the appearance of many symptoms. Its antecedents are to be found in hereditary factors, constitutional types, deviation from normal development of the skeletal frame, falls, sprains, strains, overuse of certain muscles and/or organs and underuse of others, poisons in the form of drugs, chemical additives, etc., and perhaps most important of all, faulty nutrition. These all have a cumulative effect on our physiology. (Practitioners of Eastern medicine have been saying for over two thousand years, "You're as young as your spine is healthy and flexible.")

In my practice, therefore, I treat my patients for their general health and well-being. I never replace medical therapy or treat a specific health or disease condition. Instead I try to rebalance the body chemically so it can heal itself. Most people don't understand the simplicity of health. If you put proper food into your diet and if you exercise, everything falls into place. Your body is always striving for health and wants to be well.

With each nutritional patient, I go over the crucial points in my system before we set up a program. I make sure each patient understands the principles of Biochemical Reprogramming, the basic

17

concept of acid/alkaline balance of the body, food combining, and how the digestive system works. I do not merely make mechanical corrections but also reorganize the patient's nutritional errors and, insofar as possible, correct his or her lifestyle along lines calculated to prevent or minimize the possibility of future health problems. But I want to stress right here and now that my program is designed for general health and well-being, *not* as a replacement for medical therapy nor as a specific treatment for any health or disease condition.

BIOCHEMICAL REPROGRAMMING

Biochemical Reprogramming goes far beyond "curing" disease in the conventional manner. It detects and alerts the patient to bodily predisease messages. No major organ is more important than another. Neither separate, independent, nor isolated parts of the body's organization, the organs are interdependent. The malfunctioning of one organ affects all the others. I look for the underlying causes of discomfort or disease. Then I set up an individual program to reeducate the patient, changing your taste buds, your appetite, your foods, your exercise, and your breathing habits.

In reprogramming patients we shoot for a diet that is permanently 60 to 70 percent fresh fruits and fresh vegetables but is subtly varied according to age, present physical condition, work situation (indoors or outdoors), location of residence (city or the country), marital status (happily or unhappily married, happily or unhappily single), and whether you are in your own business (you may suffer from entrepreneurial stress). I take all these variables into consideration.

ACID/ALKALINE BALANCE: THE CRUCIAL KEY TO FOOD COMBINATION

If you were my patient I would tell you that when your body is too acid, it becomes susceptible to disease. "Too acid!" you would exclaim. "What's *that?*" Then I would tell you that all bodily liquids—indeed, all liquids—are either acid or alkaline. The majority of acids that contain oxygen are known as *oxyacids*; those not containing oxygen are termed *hydrogen acids* or *hydracids*.

When the metallic elements that are present in foods are oxidized in the body, they give rise to *bases*, which are alkaline. When sulfur and phosphorus in foods are oxidized, they give rise to acids: sulfuric and phosphoric. For example, animal products, which are mainly protein, produce acid end products; fruits (even the very acid-tasting ones like lemon) produce basic, or alkaline, end products. Optimal health requires an alkaline balance.

Therefore, fruit and vegetables should predominate in the ideal diet. Fruit acids are composed of carbon, hydrogen, and oxygen and through decomposition and oxidation turn into bases, or alkalines. On the other hand, most protein decomposes and oxidizes into butyric acid, sulfuric acid, phosphoric acid, or uric acid. The body does not function properly when it is overly acidic. For a variety of well-attested medical reasons an acid imbalance weakens the body and makes it prone to disease. Remember, I am saying the *predominance* of acid-inducing foods causes disease; you may consume acid foods, but you must balance the acid with alkaline-inducing foods for optimal health.

Again, the condition and constitution of all body fluids—especially blood—is the most important factor in our health. Organs such as the kidneys, the liver, the skin, and especially the large intestine filter waste and toxins to maintain our internal environment in as ideal a condition as possible. If we eat too many acid-inducing foods, our cells eventually become unhealthy. When too many cells become sick, ill health is the result. Illness, I believe, is the body's signal that something is wrong with the internal environment and that the body has failed to correct it. Boss, do something!

When a nutritional patient comes into my office suffering from acidosis or toxicity, it is usually the result of an imbalance of acid-inducing foods. Once your body chemistry is out of synch, it is important to neutralize this condition. This is why I recommend drinking fresh-squeezed lemon juice in warm water before retiring. Lemons help cancel out the effects of eating too many acid-inducing foods during the day and restore the body's acid/alkaline balance.

You see, the acid/alkaline balance in our body fluids shifts, depending upon what we eat.

The acid/alkaline balance is measured through what we call the *pH factor*. Our bodies secrete or maintain different kinds of fluids, with different pH factors, and you will learn how I test my patients' pH—and how you can easily test your own.

I tell my patients that my program is based on the following principles:

1. To preserve the normal alkalinity of the body (the alkalinity of the blood remains a constant throughout life), you should eat 60 to 70 percent health-promoting "alkaline-inducing foods"—fresh fruits and vegetables rich in organic minerals and vitamins. This applies especially if you also eat acid-forming foods such as meat, cheese, nuts, grains. On my program you need not worry about rigid diets or calorie counting. There is no need to give up your favorite acid-forming foods. Just select them judiciously and in correct balance, and you will feel great.

2. The healthy body must be nourished with predominantly *living* mineral and alkaline elements. Fresh juicy fruits should predominate at breakfast, with occasional cereals. For lunch, fresh fruit or vegetables along with a dairy product, nuts, soups, or sandwiches. At dinner eat vegetables, especially salads. Protein foods such as poultry, fish, or meat can be eaten either at lunch or dinner. (For more information about food combining, see chapter 5.)

Be Conscious of Your Acid/Alkaline Balance
Instead of Your Calorie Intake

To be sure you stay well, plan your meals to follow the valuable acid/alkaline chart on pages 23–24. Don't get hysterical, just observe it in a rational manner. You can eat an all-acid meal, but make your next two or three meals mostly alkaline. The acid/alkaline balance in your body for optimal health is pH 7.0. Your urine should be between 6.0 and 6.5; your saliva, 7.0. By taking a pH count at the onset of treatment and at various points during the treatment, we have a barometer to gauge the success of the healing process. For instance, a young woman in her twenties complained of "cystic breasts." When I tested her pH balance, both her urine and saliva was high on the acid side—5.0, when she should have been around 6.5 or 7.0. After I put her on a heavily alkaline program of fruits and vegetables, her pH count moved up to 6.5 in a month, and the cysts shrank.

The pH factor is a crucial gauge of your body's toxicity. How do I use it? How can you use it? In developing a program for a highly acidic patient I stress more alkaline foods; for a relatively nonacidic patient I stress fewer alkaline foods. In other words, in most cases, the sicker you are, the more you need an alkaline diet. The goal should be 6.5–7.0.

Oh, no! What's this all about? Some patients become alarmed when I explain the acid/alkaline balance, thinking (and sometimes saying), "Oh, God, do I need a graduate degree in chemistry to understand this?" Don't worry. To understand, all you need think about are two familiar examples: You may not be a farmer, but you probably know that before the farmer plants his crop in the spring he takes out his little test kit to check the soil. What's he doing? He's checking the pH balance! If the soil is too acidic, he *feeds* it by adding lime to bring it up to 7.0; if the soil is too alkaline, he adds sulfur to bring it down to 7.0. Why does he do this? Simply because if the soil is *too* acid or too alkaline, his crop won't grow healthily. And when the swimming pool owner wants to check the acidity of the pool water (a once-a-week must), he goes through the same procedure. If the water is too alkaline, algae grow like crazy.

How You Can Test Your Own pH Balance

What has all this got to do with you? You can check the pH balance of your body by dipping a two-inch strip of Nitrazene paper into your saliva and another into your urine. (Both are necessary to get an accurate reading.) In only a few seconds, the paper will turn a color that you can match to one of seven shades indicating your acid/alkaline balance. You can buy this inexpensive paper in any drugstore. Similar to a thermometer or a scale, the pH check is a way of monitoring your body's health.

Be sure you do this at night before retiring (before brushing your teeth) and also in the morning right after you wake up (before brushing your teeth). (If you check after a meal, the pH simply reflects the food you've just eaten.)

A More Rational Diet Designed for the Times

The acid/alkaline chart on pages 23–24 is the key to a rational, scientific diet. It is important for you to know that once you change your diet to more alkaline-forming foods, you will probably do beautifully for a while. Then for no apparent reason you may slide downhill again, and your urine and saliva test acidic. This is due to the sloughing off of highly acidic internal wastes and toxic materials in the body. Don't worry if you have ups and downs, because you are absolutely headed in the right direction. You should feel encouraged, the diet is working. All dietary changes should be gradual, depending upon where the problem is: the liver, the gallbladder, the stomach, the intestines, the pancreas, the endocrine system.

IMPORTANT POINTS TO REMEMBER

- All protein foods are acid-forming.
- All other listed foods are alkaline.
- Eat only when hungry.
- Do not overeat.
- Do not eat when in pain or emotionally upset.
- Eat foods at room temperature.
- Do not eat when tired or immediately after hard work.
- Do not eat a meal fit for a truck driver if you are a steno.
- Eat juicy foods prior to concentrated foods.
- Eat raw foods before cooked foods.
- Exceptions:
     Apple may be combined with any vegetable in small amounts.
     Avocado may be combined with anything.
  Tomato may be combined with anything except sweet fruit and melon.
  Lettuce (preferably romaine) is permissible with fruits.

FOOD COMBINING CHART

	PROTEIN →	STARCH	FAT	NON-STARCHY VEG.	RAW GREEN VEGETABLE	ACID FRUIT	SUB-ACID FRUIT	SWEET FRUIT (DRIED)	MELON
Protein →	bad	bad	bad	good	good	poor	bad	bad	bad
Starch	bad	good	good	good	good	bad	fair	poor	bad
Fat	bad	good	good	good	good	good	good	good	bad
Green Veg.	good	good	good	good	good	poor	fair	poor	bad
Sub-Acid Fruit	bad	bad	good	poor	poor	good	good	good	fair
Acid Fruit	bad	bad	good	fair	fair	good	good	bad	fair
Sweet Fruit	poor	poor	good	poor	poor	poor	good	good	fair
Melons	bad	bad	bad	bad	bad	bad	bad	fair	good

ACID/ALKALINE CHART

SWEET FRUIT	ACID FRUIT	PROTEIN	NON-STARCHY VEGETABLES	GREEN VEGETABLES
Banana (ripe)	Cranberry	Animal foods (all)	Artichoke	Lettuce
Breadfruit	Currant	Avocado	Bamboo	Green pepper
Carob	Grapefruit	Cheese	shoot	Celery
Date	Kiwi	Chick-peas	Beans (green)	Spinach
Fig	Kumquat	Coconut	Bok choy	
Prune	Lemon	Corn (raw)	Broccoli	
Raisin	Lime	Dairy products	Brussels	
Sapote	Loganberry	Legumes	sprouts	
Dried fruit	Loquat	Lentils	Cabbage	
	Orange	Millet	Cauliflower	
SUB-ACID FRUIT	Pineapple	Nut seeds (except	Celery	
Apple	Pome-	chestnuts)	Chard	
Apricot	granate	Olives	Chicory	
Blackberry	Strawberry	Peanut butter	Chives	
Cactus fruit	Tamarind	Soybeans	Collards	
Cherimoya	Tangerine		Cucumber	
Cherry	Tomato		Eggplant	

ACID/ALKALINE CHART (Con't)

Elderberry		STARCH	Endive
Gooseberry	MELON	Banana squash	Escarole
Grape	Watermelon	Beans (lima)	Kale
Guava	Muskmelon	Beet	Kohlrabi
Huckleberry	Honey dew	Carrot	Lettuce
Jujube	Casaba	Chestnut	Okra
Mango	Canteloupe	Corn	Parsnips
Mangosteen	Banana	Grains (except	Pepper
Muleberry	melon	millet)	(sweet)
Nectarine	Cranshaw	Hubbard squash	Rutabaga
Papaya	melon	Jerusalem arti-	Sorrel
Pawpaw	Christmas	choke	Sprouts
Peach	melon	Pasta	(mung
Pear	Persian	Peas	bean, al-
Persimmon	melon	Potato	falfa)
Plum	Nutmeg	Pumpkin	Squash
Quince	melon	Rice (brown)	(except
Raspberry		Yam	starchy)
			Tomato
			Turnip
			Watercress

THE DIGESTIVE SYSTEM

Now I'll explain why poor eating habits create disease over a period
of time. Under normal conditions the digestive tract (see diagram
on opposite page) is an efficient assembly line for breaking down
and processing food so that it can pass into the bloodstream and
nourish our cells. Today it is probably the seat of most of our acute
and chronic ailments. The foods we eat, how they are combined,
and yes, even *how we chew* either help or hinder this process. All
foods must be broken down before they can pass through the walls
of the small intestine and into the bloodstream. Everything we eat
has to be reduced before it can be utilized by the body cells, a
process called *metabolism*. Now we'll examine the rest of the digestive process to show how poor nutrition *actively* breeds poor health.

The essential substances in the digestive juices that promote
the biochemical breakdown of food are called *enzymes*. These are
complex proteins that induce biochemical changes in other substances. Each enzyme breaks down a single specific substance. For
example, an enzyme that breaks down fats does not break down
proteins or carbohydrates. Enzymatic action originates in the sali-

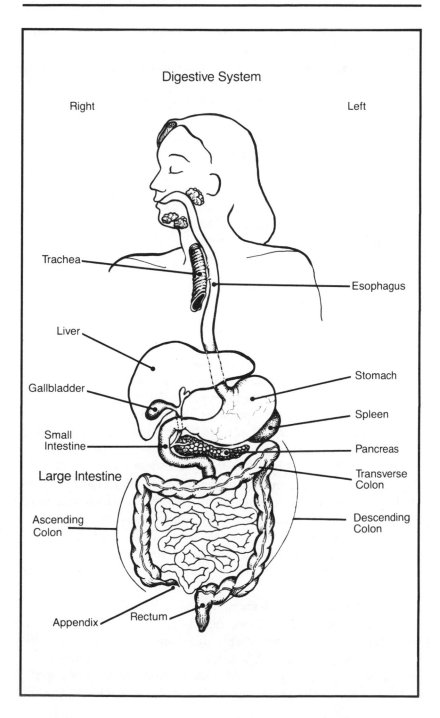

Digestive System

vary glands and continues in the stomach, liver, pancreas, spleen, and finally through the walls of the small intestine.

Nutrients, now in the form of glucose (from carbohydrates), amino acids (from protein), and fatty acids and glycerol (from fats), are absorbed by the small intestine and passed into the bloodstream. This digestive process takes place primarily in the small intestine, the lining of which is covered with small, fingerlike projections called *villi*. These villi contain lymph channels and tiny blood vessels called *capillaries*, which are the ultimate channels of absorption. Fats and fat-soluble vitamins move through the blood and lymph to every cell in your body. Other nutrients are carried away from the villi by the capillaries, which funnel them into the portal vein leading to the liver for filtering and storage.

Chew, Chew, Chew, Chew, Chew, Chew, Chew, Chew

Digestion starts in your mouth, so thorough chewing of every bit of food you put into your mouth is essential. *Indeed, it is important to eat less and chew more, rather than eat more and chew less.* Take a slice of bread. When you chew it carefully, a series of physical and chemical changes takes place. The bread is first broken down in your mouth in preparation for absorption from the intestinal tract into the bloodstream. Don't gulp it down. The salivary glands in your jaw have *ducts* (tubes) that release digestive fluids into the mouth that not only moisten food so you can swallow it easily but also convert starch and simpler sugars for easier digestion by means of the enzyme *ptyalin* (or amylase). The bread, which you have converted to liquid, slides down your esophagus on its way to your stomach. If you don't chew enough to break the food into liquid, the food, no matter how nutritious or delicious, is not absorbed or metabolized properly in your body during the rest of the digestive process.

Your stomach is predominantly acidic, and that is what helps break down proteins. Your food, including the slice of bread you've just eaten, with its carbohydrates, fats, and proteins, is partially broken down in the stomach and turned into a digestive mash.

After one to four hours, depending upon the food or combination of foods your system ingests, the *peristalstic* process pushes the bread (now in the liquid form called *chyme*) out of the stomach and through the pyloric valve into the twenty-two to twenty-six feet of your small intestine, where an important part of digestion takes place. When chyme enters the small intestine, the pancreas secretes additional enzymes that further break down the proteins and carbohydrates. If fats are present in the food (let's say you are eating a fatty pork chop), bile, an enzyme produced by the liver and stored in the gallbladder, is also added. Bile breaks down and separates the fat into small droplets so that the pancreatic enzymes can break it down still further.

The Stomach and Colon

When food enters the stomach from the esophagus, gastric juices begin to flow and the muscles of the stomach wall begin rhythmic contractions. This is the start of the process of digestion, which goes on for one to five hours. The partially digested food passes by degrees to the small intestine, where digestion continues. Food nutrients are extracted and distributed by the bloodstream to all parts of the body. The solid waste residue is now received by the large intestine (colon), where some valuable fluids are absorbed through the cecum and waste matter is passed out of the body. The colon is rectangular in shape. On the right side of the colon is your appendix, no longer considered obsolete because it has a definite lubricating effect on the colon. Your colon ends at the rectum, which narrows down to the anus. When you move your bowels, the wavelike process called peristalsis passes the debris out.

The Pancreas and Liver Are Important
Parts of the Digestive System

When your food passes from your stomach through the pyloric valve, the enzyme *enterin* signals your pancreas to release other enzymes. Alkaline enzymes go into your small intestines, where they help break down the balance of your proteins, starches, and fats. Everything else passes through the intestinal walls. Many people do not realize there is no direct connection between the intestines and the bloodstream. Solid wastes pass from the small intestine into the large intestine and are eliminated as feces. Waste liquids and nutriments both go through the walls of the small intestine into the blood. Your kidneys filter out the liquid waste and eliminate it. The nutriments go directly into the bloodstream.

Another vital organ involved in digestion is the liver, which secretes enzymes, filters out toxins, contributes to the health of the immune system, and is ultimately involved in every process in the human body. When I see a patient with muddy eyes, a pallid complexion, and foul breath, the odds are that the liver is not functioning properly.

Why Problems Start

Digestion is a complex process. Heavy smoking, heavy drinking, overconsumption of fats, and sugar addiction are only a few of the habits that not only interfere with but actively inhibit the action of the digestive system. Fresh vegetables and fruits chewed to a near liquid state are more easily digested.

Most people, however, eat conventionally, consuming huge quantities of fast foods and too many tainted animal proteins, eggs, and dairy products, all containing very little fiber. Eventually, eating these fiberless, overcooked, contaminated foods causes constipation and irritates the colon, particularly the crevices, which are called sacculations. I compare the average American colon to an encrusted pipe, in which water shoots through the middle. The colon's toxic material that hardens and solidifies is called the *fecalith* (*fecal* for fecal matter, and *lith* meaning "stone"). This impacted waste continually oozes through the permeable colon into your bloodstream, where it represents a permanent source of body pollution and ill health. In some cases, a partial cleansing such as an enema suffices; for others, I recommend an occasional colonic irrigation—a stream of lukewarm water that gently washes through the colon's valves (you are not even aware that it is happening) and cleans this whole area out. A good colonic operator (for a reputable local practitioner, ask your doctor, chiropractor, nutritionist, or health food store for a recommendation) will note the amount of undigested food or mucus in the form of hardened clumps of fecal matter that are passing through a little glass tube. This hardened waste matter may have been accumulating for fifteen to twenty years—or even longer.

Marianne, for example, suffered from colitis as a result of bad eating habits.

Marianne M.

"You're my last resort. I've been on cortisone, predni-
solone, and Valium for so many years. The side effects of
the medication are ruining my marriage . . . and my col-
itis is getting worse despite the medication. I'm passing
blood every day. I'm losing weight and the diarrhea won't
stop. I can't keep any food down. Is there any hope?"

Marianne is a thirty-nine-year-old, five-foot-two, attractive, dark-haired executive for a major corporation who traveled extensively in her work. By the time I met her, she had been forced to resign her position because of severe intestinal problems. She weighed eighty-two pounds. Her skin was abnormally pasty. She was unable to eat without excruciating pain and was literally housebound with constant bouts of diarrhea. Top gastroenterologists in Houston, Chicago, and New York City had told Marianne and her husband there was no cure for her ulcerative colitis. They prescribed medication to alleviate the pain, but a colostomy (removal of the colon), the doctors said, was inevitable.

More often than not when patients come to me, I believe I can help. But Marianne was in such bad shape, I could not promise results. All I could say was that I would try my best, but I needed her total commitment. Of course, at this advanced stage of her condition her nervous system was affected, and she burst into tears, crying uncontrollably during our first interview.

When I asked Marianne about her diet, she told me the old familiar horror story, although in her opinion she ate very well. I hear it over and over. Animal protein twice a day, and always the "best." Both she and her husband were gourmet cooks. Her highly spiced diet was rich in pastries, bakery breads, imported cheese, Godiva chocolates, and Häagen-Dazs ice cream—only the best. Marianne's digestive system could not handle this diet, and it was obvious to me that her diet was largely responsible for her problems. Now at an advanced stage, unable to keep anything else down, she was existing on farina and cream of wheat: commercial, refined cereals that only made matters worse. These cereals had very little in them beyond calories. Everything nutritious had disappeared in the manufacturing process. By the time Marianne came to see me, she was barely able to handle even this refined cereal.

My first step was to put Marianne on a natural, unrefined cereal—"rice cream," that is, a form of brown rice—which she ground down into baby-food consistency. After she was able to assimilate the rice cream, I gradually introduced into her diet other foods in the following order: thoroughly steamed vegetables, then lightly steamed vegetables, then raw vegetables, then skinless baked potatoes, then baked potatoes with the skin. Within five weeks I had her eating foods rich in vitamin A to heal the damaged soft tissue: yams, mashed carrots, lightly steamed carrots, grated carrots, yellow squash. (At Marianne's stage, raw fruits and vegetables were inadvisable. They could impact on the colon and irritate scar tissue formed through the colitis.) Since intestinal problems such as Marianne's colitis are a form of pellagra—a disease caused by a deficiency of B vitamins in the diet and characterized by skin changes, nerve dysfunction, and diarrhea—I recommended a limited course of non-yeast vitamin B supplements until her body was sufficiently healed.

Within a few weeks of eating properly combined food, the pain and diarrhea subsided. As her symptoms began to clear, her doctor gradually took her off the medication. It's now several years later, and Marianne is again a corporate decision maker. Her diet is the Long Life Diet (see chapter 5), with occasional lapses at restaurants or parties. She still comes in to see me for reevaluations. After her last visit she told me, "Dr. Soltanoff, I have never before experienced such energy, vitality, vibrance, and clarity of mind."

An interesting spin-off was the effect on Marianne's husband. When he saw the immediate results, he realized that it was crazy to go on eating in the old way and he went on my program, too. The results? An immediate surge in energy and stamina.

In Marianne's case, poor diet gave her severe chronic abdominal pain and chronic diarrhea and turned her into a walking skeleton. In Peggy L.'s case, bad diet had altogether different effects.

Peggy L.

*"I'll try anything, and I've got to start now. I know I can
be a bitch on wheels, but I don't know why. Everybody
says, 'Knock some of the weight off, and you'll feel terrific.' "*

Peggy L. was a forty-year-old, hefty, aggressive night worker
in a supermarket. At five feet nine inches, she weighed close to 250
pounds. She had been diagnosed as epileptic eleven years earlier
and since that time had been on Dilantin and phenobarbital. Her
blood pressure was 240/120, and she had been on medication for
that condition as well. Her father had died of a blood-pressure-
induced disease, and there was a family history of heart trouble and
high blood pressure. Suffering also from endometriosis, she was
slated for a hysterectomy. Her thyroid gland was sluggish, and her
pituitary gland was malfunctioning as a consequence of years on
the Pill.

Peggy's health dossier revealed twenty-eight current problems.
To balance her badly damaged body, I insisted she include sea plants
in her diet, mostly kelp and dulse (see pages 204–206). I managed
to get her walking regularly, biking on a stationary bicycle, and
rowing on a rowing machine. Peggy started systematically doing
the health and body brushing technique. She really went all out. As
her thyroid gland started to function normally, a whole chain reaction
was set off: The other glands began to work in harmony, and she
lost weight. The brushing got her circulation going. She no longer
complained about cold hands and feet and fatigue.

Still, for all her enthusiasm, Peggy was a problem patient.
Particularly in the beginning, she would go off the diet and binge
on pizza and hot dogs. I didn't browbeat her. There was no point
to that. I said, "Not to worry; just get back on the program and get
back soon." Gradually over the months those perverted taste buds
of hers were transformed. To her own amazement she lost her
craving for pizza, hot dogs, and coffee. She could not believe it.
But I told her her body had been rebalanced and it no longer had
the taste for these unnatural foods.

MOST PROBLEMS SEEM TO RELATE
TO A MALFUNCTIONING LIVER

Most problems within the digestive tract—certainly in the people I see—manifest in the liver. The liver processes the fat in our diets, and most Americans consume too much fat in foods. Fatty foods lower the oxygen available to the body by 20 to 25 percent, interfering with the circulation of blood through capillaries. In addition, they reduce all the mineral reserves in your body; fat binds up all minerals, especially calcium and magnesium, passing them right out of your body in the same way that mineral oil (often taken for constipation) leaches out vitamins A, D, E, F, and K. The result is a dangerously overworked liver.

The liver, dissected and examined by thousands of medical students and scientists over the years, is the largest of our glands. It weighs from three to four pounds. The chemical factory of the body, it has hundreds of vital duties. For example, it manufactures bile to aid fat digestion. Bile is stored in the gallbladder, which is attached to the liver. The liver is also a filter that cleans the blood of waste matter and poisons, and changes sugar into glycogen, a starch. It stores this excess sugar until needed by the body and prevents too much blood from flooding the heart. The liver also forms urea, the main element of urine, which is carried by the blood to the kidneys.

Uric acid, an ash that builds up in the urine, deserves an explanation. If you burn your rug, you'll have one kind of ash. If you burn wood, you'll have a different kind of ash. If you burn your dress or trousers, it's still another kind of ash. When you eat fruit or vegetables, an alkaline ash is usually left over; when you eat something that's derived from an animal source—fowl, fish, meat, eggs, cheese—the ash that's left over is mostly uric acid. Up until age thirty-five or forty, your four organs of excretion—lungs, skin, kidneys, bowels—eliminate the uric acid efficiently. But if one of these eliminative organs slows down (as they tend to do after age forty), it places a burden on the other three. They can't handle the overload, so uric acid is retained in the body. A liquid, it circulates in the bloodstream and gradually weakens and irritates the body. Eventually it hardens and solidifies, causing pain. The blood becomes toxic and thicker and has trouble getting through the cardiovascular system. This increases the burden on the heart and sometimes elevates blood pressure. The uric acid collects and eventually builds up in the joints as a sharp, crystalline irritant. That's how most types of arthritis form.

Though a great deal is written about the heart, kidneys, and stomach, comparatively little is known by most people in the street about the liver and its functions. Of all its hundreds of functions, the primary function of the liver is to act as a filter. It filters out poisons. As noted before, it is the chemical factory in the body, and a great many of the enzymes that break down food are manufactured in the liver. It not only filters out chemical additives and wastes, it filters out impurities or toxins that may result from cooking, baking, and pasteurization. When the liver is under severe daily stress, like any part of your body, it slows down and starts to malfunction. A first step toward improving liver function is to drink distilled water, which acts as a solvent and purifier (see page 224).

The Liver and Vitamins

When the liver becomes strained and overworked, several of its important functions are altered. For example, the liver should be able to break down and assimilate fatty vitamins A, D, E, F, and K. If it doesn't function well, however, you can take vitamin supplements from now until doomsday, and the supplements won't work. New patients come into my office with bags filled with supplements. (Some take over a hundred supplements a day!) For example, one patient, Ed, complained of night blindness (reduced vision at night) and photophobia (inability of the eyes to adjust from light to dark), and yet Ed had been taking vitamin A for four years. But I could see from his questionnaires that the problem was his liver, not his eyes. I put him on a course of Biochemical Reprogramming. After several months his liver began to function properly. Now he was able to properly assimilate vitamin A. The night blindness and photophobia gradually disappeared.

Without a properly functioning liver and the enzymes it produces, nutrients cannot get to the cells. The reactions in the liver produce the products needed by individual cells. Some of the products are used by the liver itself, but others, such as glycogen, are held in storage by the liver, to be released into the body as needed. The remainder go into the bloodstream, where they are picked up by the cells and put to work. Water-soluble vitamins, on the other hand, such as B and C and minerals, are also absorbed into the bloodstream through the walls of the small intestine (osmosis).

After Years of Abuse, Your Liver May Grow Sluggish in Middle Age

In middle age, between the ages of forty and fifty-five, most people exercise less and continue to eat and to drink as they did when they were younger and far more active. So the liver, which thrives on exercise, grows sluggish. This may cause headaches, spots before the eyes, fatigue, or a general feeling of misery and malaise, and sufferers begin to wonder whether life is worth living. These attacks are apt to come without warning. Without adequate exercise and a proper diet, even teetotalers can develop a sluggish liver. A bad diet does not need alcohol to do its damage. You cannot consistently abuse your liver and maintain your health any more than you can abuse your heart or stomach.

Here is a list of some of the liver's most important functions:

• Breaks down nitrogen into urea so the kidneys can process it.

• Stores vitamins needed by the red blood cells that manufacture marrow in the bones.

• Balances the sex hormones.

• Converts amino acids into albumen, which regulates the balance of salt and water.

• Secretes bile, which governs much intestinal activity, promotes the digestion of fats, and helps prevent us from being poisoned by alcohol or too much animal protein.

• Regulates blood clotting.

• Filters out excessive drugs, medicines, and harmful industrial chemicals.

• Enables the body to use the energy in food, stores the excess in the form of fat, converts it into glycogen, and when needed, transforms it into glucose and releases it.

The liver will break down under nutritional stress, lack of exercise, and heavy drinking. Beginning with gas and indigestion, the whole body will suffer progressively. Conversely, rest, exercise, and the right kind of food—depending on the disease—and the temporary use of vitamins tend to quickly restore the liver to health. It is a happy fact that the liver will partially regenerate itself from almost any stage of degeneracy. It is the only organ with that capacity.

What Happens to the Liver When You Eat Fatty Foods?

When you eat fatty foods, your hypothalamus, the part of the brain that contains centers controlling body temperature, thirst, hunger, water balance, and sexual function, signals your gallbladder to contract. When your gallbladder contracts, it squeezes out the bile, the enzyme manufactured by the liver that breaks down fatty foods. Most of this enzyme goes into your stomach, but some goes into your small intestine, where it helps break down the fatty particles into even smaller particles so your body can assimilate them. However, if you're eating too much fatty food (animal protein and dairy products are the prime culprits), the liver is overburdened and grows sluggish. A sluggish liver won't filter waste efficiently, so some waste collects in your bile and eventually builds up in your gallbladder in the form of gallstones. How does this come about? As an analogy, think of the oil in your car. When you put the oil in, it's a pure golden liquid, but when you drain it, the oil is a totally different substance—black, thick, and gritty with waste and debris. That's what happens to your bile. Improper diet fills your bile with waste, grit, and debris. Initially this takes the form of a "gravel" sediment. But if you persist with your improper diet, the gravel will eventually build up into stones.

Breathing Is Also a Factor in the Proper Working of Your Liver

Proper breathing massages the liver as a natural consequence of its action. But shallow breathing is a factor in a malfunctioning liver, since it fails to give the liver the continuous massage it needs to keep fit. A person cannot live for more than a few weeks without food, less than a week without water, but no more than a few minutes or so without air. Yet this most vital life support system is one of the most abused and neglected. Proper breathing oxidizes the blood, is a critical part of metabolism, and invigorates internal organs. You are a living furnace, and you burn your food through the way you breathe. (See Chapter 4.)

Today's constricting clothes are not so very different from the tightly laced corsets that women wore in the earlier days of my practice. This self-imposed torture in the name of fashion impedes proper breathing and will eventually affect normal liver function.

To sum it up, most liver and gallbladder troubles are caused by overeating and drinking; by foods that are too refined or too rich; by lack of exercise; by shallow breathing; by lack of vitamins, minerals, and enzymes; and by inadequate supply of nerve force from the spinal cord to the liver, which is often remedied by osteopathy or chiropractic. The liver needs plenty of fresh green vegetables and fruits for an adequate supply of minerals to keep it healthy.

How to Avoid Surgery

Many people suffer from gallstones, kidney stones and bladder stones. The usual prescription has always been surgery, though today lasers are taking over as the preferred technological fix. But these brutal methods can be avoided. These conditions are invariably caused by overacidity, generalized toxicity, and altered body chemistry. Consequently, to circumvent surgery as well as laser or other high-tech methods, what you have to do is bring your body back to its normal biochemical balance. Gradually the stones will disintegrate and pass out of the system. Surgery and the laser should be reserved for last-ditch emergency situations. (If the gallstones have become too large, surgery will be necessary.) Meanwhile, if you're suffering from early symptoms, the idea is to bring your body back into balance before emergencies can develop. You can embark on other strategies, beginning with a short water fast of from one to three days, during which the liver and digestive organs are rested. Then meals must be cut down to two moderate ones each day. Fats must be reduced to a minimum, and chocolate, coffee, tea, alcoholic and carbonated beverages, and chocolate-based drinks are all taboo.

NOTE: Fresh fruits and vegetables, one of the mainstays of my diet under normal circumstances, should be eaten sparingly and chewed to a near liquid state or blended by people with gallbladder problems. All dairy products including yogurt should be avoided until the condition has cleared up. Apples, nuts, and seeds should be cut out of the diet or reduced drastically. On the other hand, the citrus fruits—lemons, limes, pineapple, oranges, and grapefruit—are all excellent for liver and gallbladder problems. All fresh fruit juices (except apple), as well as all vegetable juices, are fine. Eat vegetables and fruits other than citrus lightly steamed.

Shauna R.

"Oh, Dr. Soltanoff, my body's such a mess. I've not been myself for a long spell. . . . A few years ago during a bout with amoebic dysentery, doctors put me on a fiberless diet, which I'm afraid has rather ruined my intestines. . . . Well, Dr. Soltanoff, I'll try it your way for two years. I'm a long-term person, and once I decide on a program, I do stick."

Shauna R., a remarkably independent, intelligent seventy-five-year-old Englishwoman, taught economics at the University of London before her retirement. When I met her, she was in the States on a lecture tour of American universities. More than Shauna's intestines were ruined. After filling out my questionnaires—Shauna took two days to complete them—she sent them in. When I analyzed the material, the trouble lay where I suspected: in her liver, her pancreas, her circulation, her spine. Her body was indeed breaking down because she wasn't refueling it properly. When I told her she must avoid tea, coffee, alcohol, and meat, and limit eggs, butter, and bread, she fell silent. Many new patients grasp eagerly at a new, even difficult, routine in the pursuit of optimal health—or at least loss of discomfort and pain—but not Shauna. Terribly depressed at the prospect of giving up the foods she loved, Shauna said she would "muse upon it" and call me with her decision. Two days later she walked into my office, saying she would proceed.

And proceed she did. Three weeks later, after starting on the program I prescribed, Shauna called in to say, "Dr. Soltanoff, I can't believe it, but I already feel the benefit."

I saw Shauna several times during the next three months and then once a year on her visits to the States. Except for one spell in which she succumbed to conventional eating during a lecture tour, she was letter perfect in her "healing behavior." She showed me the diary she had started, "A New Healthy Life," and I flipped the pages. Here are a few of the entries:

6/3/77
Will go off the diet very soon because of lectures at the University of Albuquerque and L.A. Am not known at these universities, will stay with friends and don't want them to think I'm strange.

6/20/77
Dr. Jack wants me to be completely vegetarian—no fish, few eggs, no meat, no chicken, no milk. So hard because growing up on a farm in England, I have come to believe fresh butter, fresh eggs, fresh milk are the best foods in the world.

8/3/78
The skin brushing is great. I've taken to it like a duck takes to water. My seventy-five-year-old skin feels and looks almost like a thirty-five-year-old skin.

7/19/80
Three years since I first saw Dr. Jack. He told me yesterday, 'You're not assimilating enough protein.' Adds a little fish, poultry, and four egg yolks a week. Try to eat

for breakfast many foods I ought to have: three dried apricots and currants for copper and iron. Lunch—big salad with one or two soft-boiled eggs (yolks only). Dinner—fish about four times a week at home in England. Must tell Dr. Jack I won't cook chicken for myself unless I can get the real free-range chicken. Healing process slow. Went through a too-thin, draggy period. And then I started to feel well again after he put me back on some animal protein.

Closing the diary, I smiled and asked Shauna if she exercised. She told me she exercised a lot. When she is in Florida, she swims about six or eight laps twice a day and walks at least two miles a day. "Try for four miles," I told her. She said she noticed her thinking was clearer. ("I was sort of dim and dour and dizzy after I retired, but after you gave me the idea of being responsible for my own body, I put myself right when I possibly can. I feel wonderful. I feel I have been given ten years of extra life.")

Although liver problems (as in Shauna's case) generally begin in middle age, even a three-year-old child may have difficulty assimilating fatty foods, such as milk and dairy products.

Rochelle N.

"Dr. Soltanoff, I'm really at the end of my tether. My three-year-old daughter Ellen has been suffering from recurring and excruciating earaches. I went to a well-known ear, nose, and throat specialist in Manhattan, but I'm not so sure he knows the answer either. I'm not a doctor, but it seems to me that something Ellen is eating is making her sick. But when I asked my specialist about it, he just laughed at me. 'What are you, a health food nut?' he scoffed. 'Where do you get your information from, Reader's Digest? You're killing your child. Her tonsils and adenoids have to come out. If she doesn't have surgery at once, she'll go deaf.' "

By the time she came to see me, Rochelle N., a thirty-five-year-old makeup artist from New York City, had been to a series of ear, nose, and throat specialists for her daughter Ellen. She had also been reading up on nutrition on her own. She had heard about my program through friends. Meanwhile, little Ellen was in bad shape following a series of severe colds, throat infections, and earaches. Even so, Rochelle, who had had a bad experience of her own with surgery, wanted to avoid it with Ellen if possible.

Was Ellen on medication? Yes, of course. Lots of it. Rochelle told me Ellen was so medicated she was constantly sleepy. As I recall, she said Ellen was "knocked out like a zombie." I asked Rochelle if her daughter drank milk.

"Of course. Four glasses of chocolate milk a day."

"Take her off milk right away." Most children can't digest cow's milk, I told her.

"What about her calcium?"

I told Rochelle that the calcium-only-from-milk propaganda was so much hooey. I am not really setting out to put the dairy farmers out of business, and I do think all farmers deserve to make a living. There is something wrong about a society where the small farmer can't make a living. But the fact remains—and it's a well-known fact—that a lot of people, especially children, can't digest cow's milk. Period! Lots of kids are actually allergic to it, and it seemed to me altogether likely that little Ellen was one of these.

I told Rochelle to eliminate all dairy products from Ellen's diet and to give her fresh juice, fruits, and vegetables. Sure enough, within a month or so, little Ellen's ear, nose, and throat problems totally disappeared. And they never returned! I hope that Rochelle and Ellen spent the money that would have gone into the surgeon's new Mercedes on a holiday for themselves.

This is a good place to say a little bit more about milk and its total nonnecessity in the adult and even children's diet. We can take our cue from the animal kingdom. What animal drinks milk after the weaning stage? None! And that is how much *we* need milk. In my opinion, dairy products are the biggest single cause of hardening and narrowing of the arteries, arthritis, respiratory ailments, digestive and skin problems. I apologize to the dairy industry and hope they start growing organic vegetables instead.

So where do you get your calcium? Broccoli, corn, oatmeal,

sesame seeds, most raw nuts, especially almonds, millet, molasses, dates, kelp, dulse, and all green leafy vegetables.

The Problems: Overeating, Assimilation, and Absorption

You can be eating the best food in the world, but if more food is being taken into your body than can be efficiently utilized, digested, assimilated, and absorbed into the bloodstream, you are overloading your entire body. In other words, fats, carbohydrates (which are sugars and starches), and proteins must be metabolized through different systems. Overeating or eating the wrong combinations of these foods especially overstresses the endocrine system, which regulates your internal metabolic environment.

Too much food is one problem; too-rich food is another. Various diseases can be triggered by food that is too rich. For example, diabetes can be caused by too much sugar or refined carbohydrates. Oleomargarine, synthetic fats, and commercial mayonnaise will in the long run contribute to hardening of the arteries. Today the food industry adds aluminum and plastics (you don't believe it?—just read those labels!) to most "natural" "pure" margarine and synthetic fats. (Aluminum compounds cause constipation and have been associated with Alzheimer's disease.)

You can get fat just by eating food that is too rich. You can also get gout and arthritis. This is what happens. Excess undigested food is carried into the intestinal tract in the form of toxic substances or poisons. The fats then become rancid, the starches ferment, and the proteins putrefy. Technically this is called *intestinal toxemia*. Practically it means you're on the road to chronic disease of one sort or another. The message: Too rich is as bad as too much. Don't overload your body on a regular basis.

Let me tell you about Kim, a confessed sugar "junkie" before she was diagnosed as having multiple sclerosis.

Kim B.

"I had pins-and-needles feelings in my legs, and I saw a neurologist almost five years ago, who diagnosed multiple

*sclerosis. He put me in a hospital for two weeks for tests
and physical rehabilitation. In the hospital I was in a
wheelchair, but by the time I got out a few weeks later,
I could use a walker, then crutches. Finally I was able
to walk, although the pins-and-needles feelings persisted.
Three years later I started to lose the sight in my left eye.
The neurologist diagnosed it as optic neuritis, which he
said was a symptom of multiple sclerosis. But I felt healthy,
and I thought there was something I could do.''*

A brilliant thirty-year-old blonde, Kim is an employment man-
ager for a Wall Street commodities and agribusiness corporation.
Having grown up in the town where I now live and practice, Kim
would visit her parents on weekends. One Sunday morning three
years ago, her mother drove her to my office. Even as she told me
about her problems, unusually severe in a thirty-year-old, Kim revealed determination and industriousness.

Kim's eye was getting worse, and she was afraid she was going
blind. The next day she filled out the questionnaires. The following
Sunday we had our first three-hour session, followed up by weekly
three-hour sessions for six to eight weeks. Our procedure, I told
Kim, was to find out the root of the problem and treat the ailing
organ(s). Kim's answers to the questionnaires led me to suspect the
liver.

I had Kim cut out alcohol, smoking, and her usual three or
four cups of coffee a day. She didn't want to—nobody wants to—
but she was scared stiff, so she accepted my advice without protest.
I also put her on my health and beauty skin brushing program. That
she loved. Everybody loves the brushing. I gave her breathing exercises, and we discussed her mental attitude.

Kim's symptoms were caused by deterioration of the myelin
sheath, the outer covering or insulation surrounding the axons, or
fibers, of all nerves—in Kim's case the optic nerve. Kim's malfunctioning liver was producing insufficient myelin sheathing. After
a month on my program, her body began to recover and her eyesight
quickly returned to normal. Her leg problems took longer to respond
because the damage was more severe and deeply entrenched. But
that also eventually yielded to treatment. She is now completely
well. Then there was Christine L., another junk food junkie.

Christine L.

"They told me it was juvenile diabetes and they put me on insulin injections and now they've stepped the dose up already. Each week they're giving me more. The doctors in Rochester said they thought it might be from stress because I'm getting married in two months and moving to Boston."

Christine's mother was one of my patients, and when she called me she was absolutely frightened to death. Insulin at twenty-three! She said she was sure I could do something to help her daughter. So Christine, a bright and bubbly twenty-three-year-old, drove three hundred miles across state from Rochester with her fiancé to see me. She had the classic symptoms of diabetes: blurred vision, severe headaches, leg cramps, insatiable thirst, frequent urination, and rapid weight loss, no matter how much junk food she ate and sodas she drank. The prescribed diet she was following was from my point of view a nutritional catastrophe.

I took her off dairy products, wheat, soda, and diet sodas (no percentage in giving up sugar just to take in a synthetic sweetener). I put her on distilled water and fruit juices (diluted fruit juices in the beginning, since I wasn't exactly sure what her system could handle). By fruit juice I meant fresh fruit juice—not the stuff in the can or frozen concentrate. I told her to eat fresh fruit, fresh vegetables, and millet. Diabetics often think that the sugar in fresh fruit is the same as the refined sugar in the bag. This is nonsense. It isn't. The pancreas breaks down and utilizes fruit sugar but is irritated and overstimulated by refined sugar.

Christine's problems were caused primarily by overloading on junk food. As a result, her body was excessively acid. I advised her to make one of her three daily meals just cherries. Cherries contain a substance that neutralizes uric acid in the body. If you can't get fresh cherries, buy dried cherries in a health food store. These dried cherries swell up overnight when you soak them. The soaking breaks down the fiber and makes them more easily digestible (I recommend soaking all dried fruit for this reason).

The doctor who diagnosed Christine's juvenile diabetes had initially prescribed six units of insulin, and within the same week

increased the dose to eight units. Naturally I told Christine to stay
on the insulin he had prescribed, but within three weeks on the
Biochemical Reprogramming diet I recommended, Christine's blood
sugar dropped. By the time the manuscript of this book is finished,
Christine's dosage of insulin will be down to two units every other
day (I assume she will be off insulin eventually). When I asked
Christine how she was doing, she told me it is not hard to stay on
a natural healing program when your life is at stake.

If Christine had continued taking higher and higher doses of
insulin, it might well have been fatal by the time she was thirty-
five. (I am not suggesting that anyone on insulin should stop taking
it. Unless the blood sugar drops, insulin therapy is necessary. Ke-
toacidosis, which results from a severe insulin deficiency, can be
fatal.) Establishment medicine unequivocally states that juvenile
diabetes is incurable. My view is that if it is, it is because these
kids continue eating junk foods! Nobody ever tells them otherwise.
Young people don't find it easy to exercise self-control, but Christine, fortunately, has discipline. She said she loves the skin brushing
so much, she and her fiancé brush together. Brushing helps her stay
on the diet. In Christine's case, the brushing is especially valuable
since it improves circulation. Diabetics are notoriously prone to
gangrene—one of the last stages of malfunction and pollution of
the circulatory system.

Bea R.

*"The arthritis in my hands gets more and more painful.
Sometimes it's so painful I can't sleep at night."*

Bea is a retired sixty-two-year-old food editor from Toronto.
In her professional capacity she had home-tested meats, cakes, cookies, and pies for years. Her nutritional background was official SAD
(see the Standard American Diet, pages 236–237), which is to say
she considered it "well balanced—eggs, bread, meat."

Bea came to me with excruciating arthritis, and like most arthritics, she was as stiff as a board. I was convinced the pain would
swiftly respond to moderate exercise and a strict diet of fresh foods,
while skin brushing would work wonders with the stiffness.

Sure enough, after several weeks of Biochemical Reprogramming, the symptoms were clearing up, right on schedule. But as it happened, Bea was far from an ideal patient. She wouldn't stick to the 70 percent fresh food regimen. My experience is that patients can be healed even when they refuse to take their own best interests into consideration. Bea would not keep to the diet, but she brushed and exercised faithfully. I put her on breathing exercises and nightly Epsom salt baths.

There are right and wrong ways to take Epsom salt baths for arthritis. Here is my recommendation:

How to Take an Epsom Salt Bath to Help Relieve Pain from Arthritis

Empty out a four-pound box of Epsom salts into one quarter of a tub of hot water. Immerse yourself in it, leaving the tap on a trifle in order to maintain an even temperature until the water gradually covers your body. After fifteen minutes in water as hot as you can possibly tolerate, let the hot water out and turn on cold or cool water (depending on how you can tolerate it). Stay in the full tub of cool water four minutes. After the bath, rub yourself briskly with a rough towel. Sip a glass of lukewarm water with the juice of one lemon and get into bed. This procedure enhances the quality of your sleep, as it helps break down the uric acid deposits in your joints. The following morning, eat a grapefruit for breakfast. Follow this regimen daily for the first week, on alternate days the second week, and twice weekly after that until all symptoms disappear. Within a month, most people see definite improvement. This procedure is not recommended for seriously ill, sedentary seniors or those with cardiovascular disease or hypertension. However, after consulting with their physicians, most people suffering from these diseases can do this in a modified form. Proceed with caution.

I particularly recommend one meal a day of fresh pineapple, the only fruit that contains substantial amounts of the mineral enzyme *bromelin*, which seems to have a salutary effect on most arthritic conditions because it helps dissolve those uric acid buildups in the various joints of the body. At the same time, I just as strongly disapprove of all grains except millet—and, in limited quantities, buckwheat groats and brown rice. It is the gluten in the grains that irritates the uric acid deposits that are responsible for provoking the pain and stiffening the joints. Arthritics, cut out bread!

Jennifer R.

"I thought my migraine headaches had disappeared forever, Dr. Soltanoff, but they came back and they're worse than ever."

Jennifer R., who had suffered migraine headaches that disappeared only to return a few years later due to stress, was able to help herself by helping others.

Jennifer, a forty-four-year-old childless homemaker, lived in a small Canadian town where her husband worked for a utility company. Jennifer had suffered terrible migraines for many years. Since she was not working outside the home, most of her time was devoted to coping with her headaches. She read every book in print on the subject and had consulted innumerable specialists. None of them had suggested a change in nutrition. I put her on Biochemical Reprogramming, and gradually over the course of several years, the migraines became less severe—and then disappeared completely. I heard nothing from Jennifer for two years. Then she called me with the bad news that her headaches had returned.

Was she following her diet? Yes. Was she doing her exercises? Yes. Was she brushing? Yes. This did not sound promising, and I had her come down for a reevaluation. After talking with her at some length, it became increasingly clear to me that the problem this time was emotional, not nutritional. She was going crazy with too much time on her hands and was worrying herself back into her headaches, imagining that her husband was cheating on her.

Obviously the answer to her headaches lay outside the sphere of my usual practice. In talking things over, a possible solution occurred. Jennifer had time to kill and nothing to do, but as it happened, a home for the aged had opened up near her house. On occasion she'd stop in there and talk with some of the old people. Having followed my diet for years, she was appalled at what these poor old people put through their digestive systems: white toast and coffee, processed cereal and milk for breakfast; luncheon meat for lunch; pork chops for dinner. It occurred to me to turn Jennifer into a nutritional crusader. This was something new. She had never made a speech, never tried to assert herself in any way. But the idea was appealing.

Jennifer went back to Canada full of enthusiasm—and a few qualms. As it turned out, the crusade was successful. First she convinced the owners of the home of the necessity for a more balanced diet. This change of mind had a certain economic basis —since it would involve fewer cooks and lower food costs.

But then the problem was the patients: getting these old folks to change their ways, even though it would mean more and healthier years for them. This campaign called into play all Jennifer's persuasive and creative powers. She found herself with a full-time volunteer job on her hands, she forgot about her husband's imagined infidelities, and once again the migraines disappeared.

Some Thoughts in Review

I cannot stress often enough that your body will not handle systemic overload. Too much and/or too-rich food does not get digested. These undigested food particles are turned into toxins that, through bacterial action, render the fats rancid. The carbohydrates start to ferment in the stomach, and the proteins putrefy. When these toxic end products proliferate in the intestinal tract, we have a condition known as intestinal toxemia. And sickness cannot be far behind.

For optimal health, the body requires unprocessed, untampered-with foods and foods uncontaminated by chemical preservatives. To maintain a high state of health and resistance to disease, it is essential to consume live foods rather than "foods" embalmed with chemicals and preservatives. Fast eating, overeating, insufficient chewing, wrong food combinations, eating at irregular hours, excessive use of tea, coffee, alcohol, sweets, soda, and tobacco eventually cause a disturbance in the digestive organs, producing indigestion, hyperacidity, heartburn, gas, constipation, or diarrhea.

It is easy to see how the stomach and intestines become the first seat of disease. I repeat, fresh vegetables and fruits eaten raw and chewed to a near liquid state are more easily digested than most people believe. These are the important foods that are alive and most conducive to healthful living and natural healing.

CHAPTER 3

Amazing Connections: Dr. Soltanoff's Unique Dry Brushing for Health and Beauty

The next crucial prong of my three-pronged Biochemical Reprogramming system is dry brushing. Dry brushing paves the way. It's what makes Biochemical Reprogramming different from any other program you might have heard about or tried. For the body to achieve optimal health, most body systems must be working on all eight cylinders. The skin provides the easiest access to certain of these systems, most importantly the nervous and the endocrine systems.

The key to a healthy immune system is the endocrine system. If the endocrine system functions properly, you need never grow sick, never grow "old." You see, the endocrine system, together with the central nervous system, was' designed to keep the body healthy and vigorous to an advanced age. It is improper nutrition, sedentary living, and the world's pollution that swell and toxify the glands, provoking disease. In fact, most illness is directly related to malfunctioning glands. (For more specific information, see pages 70–77.) Dry brushing stimulates the glands, promoting their return to proper function. In my opinion, it may well be the emphasis on brushing that gives such extraordinary results with my patients. When I get patients brushing, they're on cloud nine. I tell them no matter what they do (unless they are very sick indeed), even if they lapse in their diet and exercise, if they keep on brushing they are going to get results. In other words, if they do brushing alone, their health is going to improve considerably. How is this possible? Because the skin is one way of reaching the endocrine system very quickly. Let's consider the skin.

The Skin Is a Complex, Vital Organ

How many of us know much about the skin or take it into consideration when we think about our health? Usually people think of skin in a purely cosmetic sense. Skin is not supposed to get wrinkled or look old. Skin looks good suntanned, though the dangers of too much sun on skin are now generally recognized. It's something that holds us together. If we didn't have it, we would leak.

In fact, the skin is an organ—the largest eliminative organ of the body, so much so that it is sometimes called the third kidney. In the course of a day the skin eliminates more than a pound of waste products in the form of sweat. Hundreds of thousands of tiny sweat glands all over the body throw out metabolic wastes, but if the skin is inactive, stuffed into tight clothes, and swathed in synthetics, it cannot do its job. The skin needs to breathe (it's also called the third lung). It needs fresh air and stimulation. Very few of us get to expose our bodies to fresh air on a routine basis. For optimum health, your entire body should be exposed to fresh air for a minimum of ten to fifteen minutes a day. Tight clothes prevent the skin from breathing, and the use of synthetic fabrics drastically compounds the problem. It's like walking around with your body coated with Saran Wrap.

The skin is also an absorptive organ. It absorbs oxygen, vitamins, minerals, even protein. By the same token, this also means that if you routinely apply toxic substances to your skin, they are going to find their way into your internal organs. Antiperspirants, by the way, amount to skin sabotage. They prevent your skin from exercising its proper eliminative function. With proper diet, brushing, and clothes made of 100 percent cotton next to your skin, you'll never need antiperspirants again. (More on skin sabotage when we talk about cosmetics.) In more natural surroundings where people lived natural lives tied to nature and natural processes, the skin probably would take care of itself and perform its function. But in our highly unnatural environment, the skin needs special attention.

As with other organs, if the skin seriously malfunctions, it will bring down the whole system. Yet, it's amazing how, even among health and fitness conscious people, the skin is taken for granted and left to its own devices.

Good nutrition and exercise are absolutely essential for putting us back on the road to health and keeping us there. But if our skin isn't doing the job it was designed to do, we will not reap the full benefit of good nutrition and exercise. Dry brushing is 100% pleasureable. A diet, any diet, involves a certain amount of sacrifice, let's face it. No matter how much good you know it's going to do you, it's going to involve giving up some favorite sins. The same goes for exercise. Working up a sweat means just what it says— working. But dry brushing—the prescription for getting your skin back in shape—is fun. All my patients, without exception, love to brush. And some of the most incorrigible exercise haters and junk food junkies find time to brush on a daily basis.

What Dry Brushing Does—and Why It Does It

Dry brushing is based upon the ancient Chinese concepts of acupuncture and acupressure (concepts, incidentally, that have recently been acknowledged as sound by Western medicine after decades of derision and neglect). The Chinese recognize three million nerve points spread over the surface of the skin, seven hundred of which are nodal. In plain language, when these nodal points are stimulated, currents flow through channels called *meridians* and stimulate (or suppress) the activity of specific organs to which they are connected. For example, the tip of your big toe is connected to the pituitary gland just below the brain. A point in the web between the thumb and forefinger of the right hand connects to the liver. Although medical researchers still do not exactly understand the mechanisms at work in acupuncture and acupressure, it is now generally acknowledged that they *do* work.

Dry brushing is systematically designed to take advantage of these myriad connections. By applying friction to the acupuncture points, your entire nervous system is stimulated and invigorated and the beneficial effects are directly conveyed to every organ, gland, muscle, and ligament in your body. Indirectly even the production of red and white blood cells is affected.

The immediate result of a brushing session is a feeling of intense physical well-being. The quality and texture of your skin improve instantly. The skin has a warm rosy glow, and you can feel your circulation revving up. In my practice I get a lot of people in from IBM and the local newspapers who must sit in front of computer screens all day long. They come to me with their neck and shoulders rigid, tied in knots. Brushing instantly releases stress and tightness in neck and shoulders. Posture is improved, and any muscular constrictions in those areas are released, thus increasing the flow of blood from body to brain and back again. *Brushing relieves chronic tension headaches far more efficiently than do painkillers.* By stimulating the lungs (when the muscles relax, the chest opens up, freeing the lungs to expand more) and increasing the flow of oxygen to the brain, brushing leads to clearer thinking. It also improves digestion, as you burn up a good portion of the food you consume through the way you breathe. If your lungs and breathing are restricted, an additional burden is placed on the heart, which prevents it from functioning normally. The quality of your blood is also upgraded through brushing. Brushing enhances both the quantity and quality of the red blood cells, which in turn benefit your overall circulation.

Beauty Benefits Through Brushing

In women, dry brushing done regularly and in conjunction with the proper diet and moderate exercise will tone and tighten the skin and will get rid of troublesome cellulite! In ninety-nine cases out of one hundred, my women patients have reduced their accumulations of cellulite in dramatic fashion, even though they came to me with unrelated problems. Cellulite is toxic material stored in the body's fat cells that does not get eliminated as it should. Cellulite builds up through a number of factors: pollution, stress, alcohol, dairy products, coffee, and general adherence to SAD (see pp. 236–7). Brushing in combination with proper diet and exercise breaks down these fatty deposits, which are gradually released and passed out as waste. (If you're so desperate to get rid of cellulite that you contemplate liposuction surgery, try brushing before you submit to this expensive and potentially dangerous operation.) Because dry brushing also stimulates hormone- and oil-producing glands, your skin will be rosy, resilient, and youthful without recourse to dangerous and expensive hormonal creams, oils, and cosmetics. (The routine destruction of millions of helpless animals by cosmetic firms should be enough to make sensitive human beings stop using their products without further inducement. Regular brushing makes their products not only immoral but unnecessary. I'm aware, of course, that there are a number of small cosmetics firms with a conscience. These do not use animals in their tests and employ only natural ingredients in their products, and I do not mean to condemn them.)

During the transition, if your skin is dry, a quick oil massage will work wonders. As a moisturizer, use a cold-pressed natural oil. Sesame, avocado, almond or extra virgin olive oil works fine. Astonishingly, for a permanently velvet-smooth skin, the best moisturizer is the cheapest by far. There is absolutely nothing better for your skin than plain 100 percent cocoa butter or coconut oil. The best skin care in the world should not cost you more than five dollars a year.

Dry Skin Health and Beauty Dry Brushing Technique

What you need is a brush about the size of your hand with a moderately soft natural vegetable fiber bristle. (Nylon or synthetic fibers are too sharp and may hurt the skin.) I'm a chiropractor/nutritionist, not a brush salesman, but the truth is, in over forty years of brushing I have never found a brush that was absolutely ideal. But inspired by the impending publication of this book, I went to a brush manufacturer and had a brush designed to my specifications. That brush is now available and you may find it does the job. (See page 288.) But any natural vegetable fiber bristle brush you're comfortable with is fine.

Skin sensitivity varies, of course, from person to person. Maybe you can stand harder brushing than I can. Also, some parts of the body are more sensitive than others: the inner thighs, abdomen, and chest particularly. Brush gently at first. When your skin has become used to brush therapy, you may, if you like, use a coarser (even synthetic) bristle. Test for comfort by rubbing the bristles of the brush over the back of your hand. (The sensation should not be unpleasant.) Within a few days, your initially tender skin becomes conditioned. Use the brush as directed on your body. The whole process should take no more than nine minutes.

Every two weeks or so, wash your brush with soap and water and dry it in the sun or in a warm place. Your brush will rapidly fill with impurities and should be washed regularly. For hygienic reasons, each member of the family should have a separate brush.

HOW TO BRUSH

Dry brushing is best taken nude in front of a mirror when you wake up in the morning before you shower. (Remember, you and the brush must be dry to create the correct friction.) You'll soon find out it has the shot-in-the-arm effect of caffeine and jogging. After a couple of weeks brushing will be second nature. You'll brush your body as automatically as you brush your teeth. In fact, it will be unthinkable to start your day without brushing. Follow the instructions exactly (and in the proper sequence) for best results. *Note:* Do not brush if you have poison ivy, skin rashes, infections, or other skin problems, or inflammatory circulatory problems such as phlebitis. Always begin by brushing gently. *Do not overbrush to the extent of irritating your skin.*

Hands and Fingers

1. Holding your right hand with your fingers extended, brush each finger back and forth 7 times.

2. Brush the entire surface of the palm side of the hand from the wrist to the finger tips back and forth 7 times; then do the same for the top of the hand.

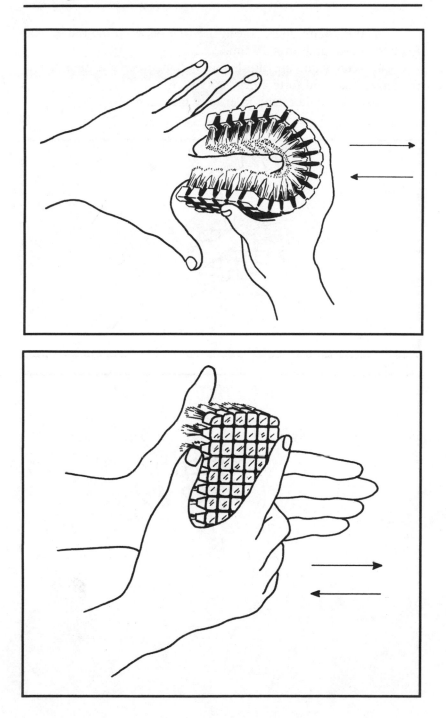

3. With palm down, brush the web between the thumb and forefinger back and forth 14 times.

4. With palm up, brush the web between the thumb and forefinger back and forth 14 times.

Now do the left hand in exactly the same way.

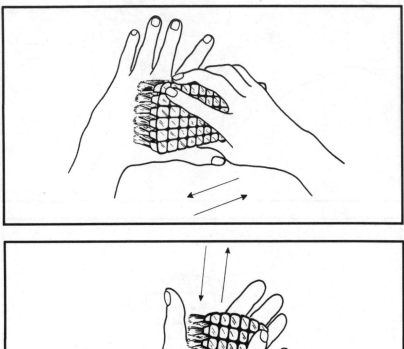

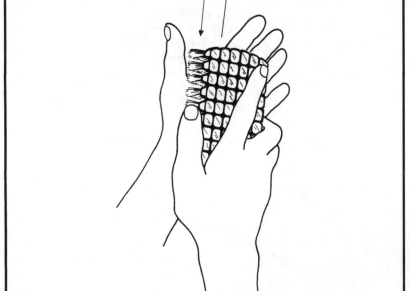

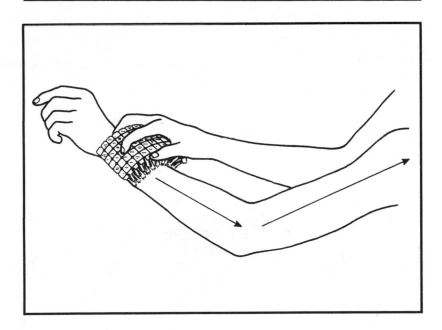

Arms

5. Brush the entire surface of the right arm from the wrist to the elbow UP towards the heart 7 times; gradually work around the entire surface of the arm doing each area 7 times. Continue from the elbow to the shoulder always UP towards the heart, again brushing each area 7 times. Repeat on left arm.

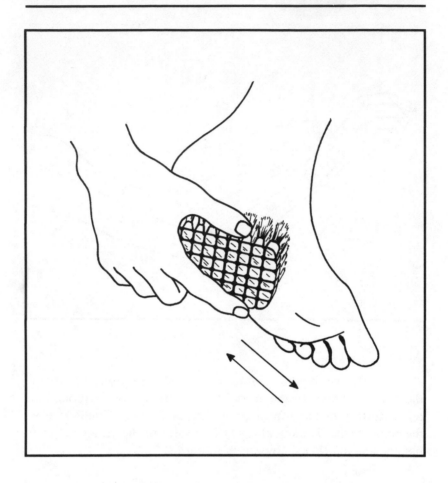

Toes, Feet, and Legs

6. Brush the entire surface of the bottom of the right foot back and forth 7 times. It'll tickle at first.

7. a. Brush across the tops of the toes back and forth 7 times. Then do the bottom of the toes.

     b. Work upward from the toes, bringing the brush *back and forth* across the top of the foot 7 times in each area up to the point at which the ankle begins.

     c. Brush around the ankles *back and forth* 7 times.

     d. Brush from the ankle to the knee UP towards the heart 7 times; gradually work around the entire surface of the leg. Don't neglect the knee area. Brushing will firm

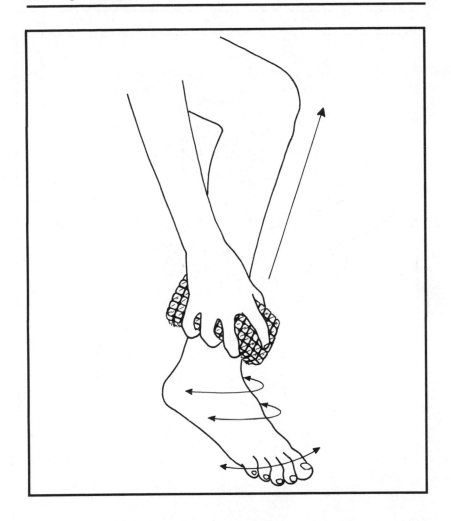

up saggy knee caps and free up congested circulation
in the back of the knee.

e. Stand and brush from the top of the knee to the hip,
always UP towards the heart, 7 times. Gradually work
around the leg so that every square inch of skin is
brushed.

Now repeat the entire procedure for the left foot and
leg.

NOTE: If you have a cellulite problem here or elsewhere,
double or treble the amount of brushing in those areas.

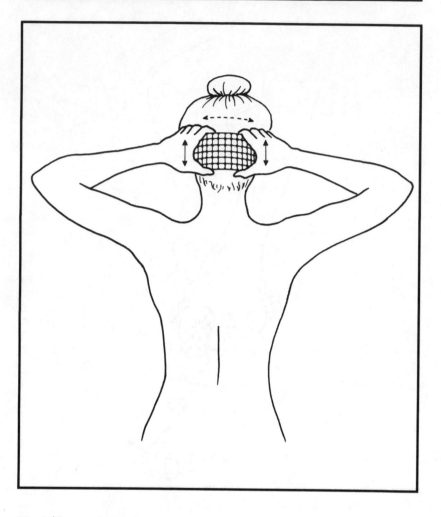

Neck/Base of Head

8. Lock brush at the base of head. *The brush should remain in place*. With two hands on the brush, rock it 14 times up and down and 14 times side to side. (This helps stimulate the pituitary gland, your master gland.)

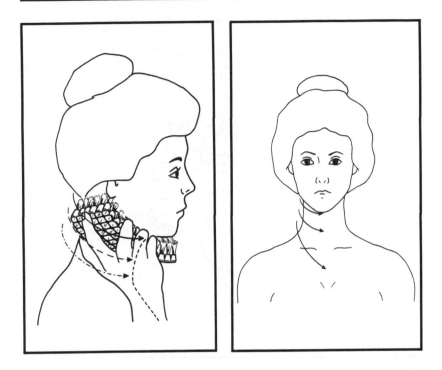

9. a. Hold the brush with your right hand, placing it under your ear on your jaw on the right side of your head. Slide it GENTLY along the jaw bone, ending by pulling through under the chin. Do this 7 times.

b. Hold the brush in your right hand at the nape of neck, then slide it GENTLY around to the right side and forward to the larynx. Do this 7 times. This helps activate the thyroid and parathyroid glands to utilize calcium.

c. Hold the brush in your right hand at the 'dowager's hump' on the top of the spine and bring the brush GENTLY around to the right and slide through the hollow of sternal notch on top of breast bone, just below the Adam's Apple. (Women: Do not brush breasts.) Do this 7 times. This stimulates the thymus gland, and will help strengthen your immune system.

Holding the brush with your left hand, do the left side of the head and neck in the same way.

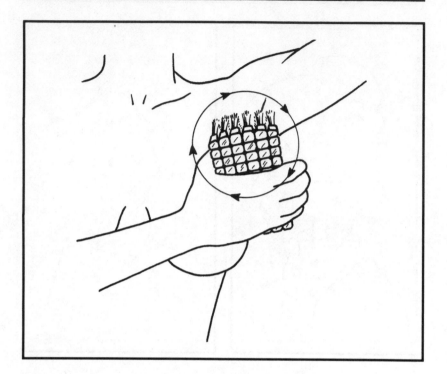

Lymphatic System (Drainage or sewage system)

10. Hold the brush firmly in the left armpit with the right hand. With the brush locked firmly in place, rotate it 7 times to the left and 7 times to the right. Then do the right armpit, using your left hand to hold the brush.

NOTE: Once you start No. 11, you stand and remain standing.

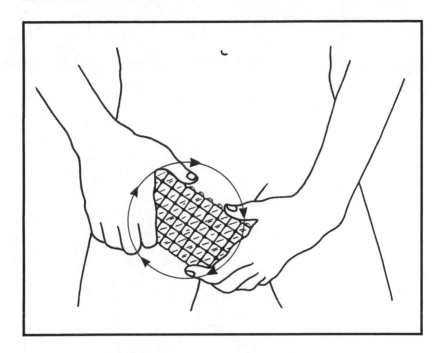

11. Hold the brush firmly in the right groin with both hands. With the brush remaining in place, rotate it 7 times to the left and 7 times to the right. Then do the left groin.

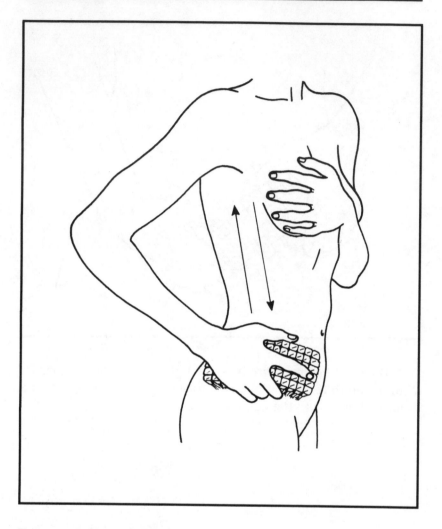

Front and Sides of Body

12. Holding the brush in the right hand, brush the right side up and down 14 times from the upper thigh all the way to under the arm. Women should hold their breast clear with the left hand out of the way of the brush. Then do the left side, using your left hand to hold the brush.

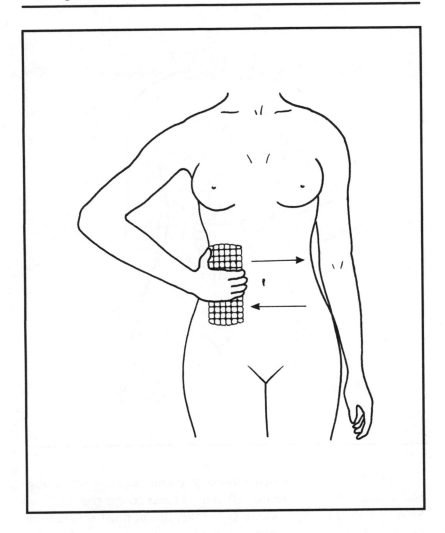

13. Brush back and forth *across and around* the waistline 14 times.

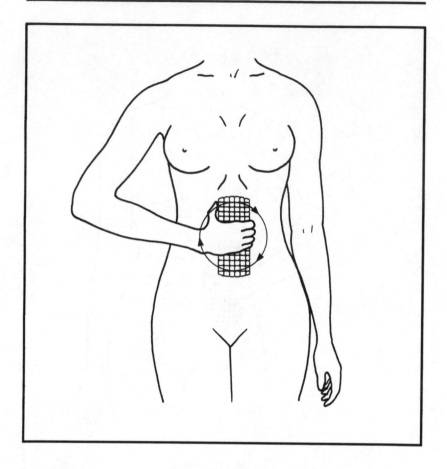

14. Brush in a circular motion at center between rib hollow (solar plexis) 14 times to the left and 14 times to the right.
Starting at the top and working all the way down, finish up the front of the body in any direction (7 times), but be sure to exclude the breasts (in women) and face since this tissue is very sensitive.

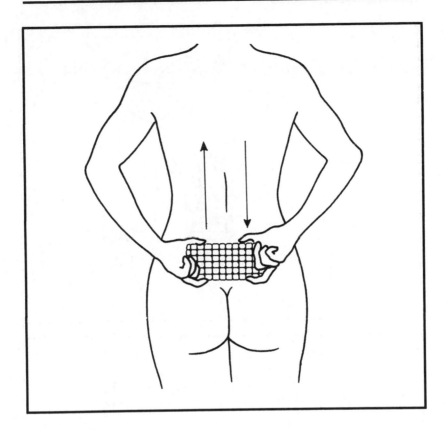

Back

15. Holding the brush with *two hands*, brush up and down 14 times along the spine starting at the coccyx (tailbone) and reaching as high as you can.

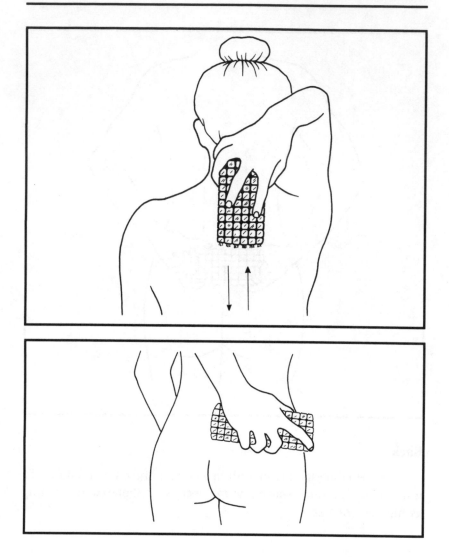

16. Holding the brush with *one hand*, brush up and down 14 times along the spine, starting at the base of neck or dowager's hump and reaching down as far as you can.
Finish the back in any direction.

17. Brush the buttocks in any direction covering the entire area 7 times. Give special attention to the buttocks and upper thighs. This will help rid the body of cellulite.
After brushing, take a shower to wash away dead skin particles.

In a surprisingly short time, a few weeks at most, you will notice that brushing contributes to healthier muscle tone, a better distribution of fat deposits, and a feeling of vigorous well-being.

The Clothing Connection

To maintain the benefits of dry skin brushing, be sure that your skin only comes into contact with natural fibers that will allow it to breathe. That means cotton underwear, cotton shirts, and especially cotton socks. For natural drainage purposes, the pores on the bottom of the feet are twelve to fourteen times larger than any other place on the body. Synthetic socks block the process. Cotton is comfortable, absorbent, entirely beneficial, and in many cases, as cheap as or cheaper than clammy polyester. I must say I can never understand how people can be so insensitive or fashion crazy that they would wear this revolting stuff next to their bodies. Nylon ski parkas, okay. But polyester blouses, no thanks! Your bed sheets should also be cotton. The poly blends do not absorb the way cotton does. In other words, the sweat stays on you. For the well-heeled and luxury-loving, pure silk sheets and undergarments also do the job.

Health and Beauty Benefits of Dry Brushing

- Stimulates and increases blood circulation in all organs and tissues, especially capillaries near the skin. Especially valuable to the over-fifties, who commonly experience cold hands and feet resulting from clogged capillaries.
- Stimulates the eliminative capacity of the skin, helping it to rid the system of toxins, placing less of a burden on the kidneys, lungs, and colon.
- By stimulating nerve endings in the skin, rejuvenates the entire nervous system.
- Drastically reduces cellulite deposits—notoriously unresponsive to other forms of treatment.
- Tones and tightens skin.
- Improves your general overall health. Helps prevent premature aging and increases resistance to colds.
- Improves clarity of thought. By stimulating the lungs and

increasing oxygen to the brain, brushing actually improves thinking.
• Often relieves chronic headaches without recourse to pain-killers.

How the Connections Work

As I mentioned earlier, the dry brushing program stimulates the endocrine and other systems. When you understand the technical formal relationships between the three prongs of the program and your various glands and organs, you'll be much more inclined to practice the program because you'll see that it's rooted in science rather than personal opinion.

The Endocrine System

The endocrine system (see diagram, p. 71) is made up of glands. The glands secrete or generate hormones that go directly into the blood. The distinction between glands and organs is not generally understood. The organs function directly, actively; for example, the heart pumps, the kidneys filter, the liver stores, the lungs breathe, the stomach digests. The endocrine glands, on the other hand, regulate. The hormones are like traffic cops, instantly dispatched to various parts of the system to control and direct innumerable bodily activities. The manner in which tiny amounts of these specific substances target in on their destination and perform their delicate and complex tasks is one of the great mysteries and miracles of creation. The endocrine system includes the pineal gland, pituitary gland, thyroid and parathyroid glands, thymus, adrenals, pancreas and islets of Langerhans, testes (male), and ovaries (female).

The Pineal Gland

The pineal gland is a tiny cone-shaped gland buried between the lobes of the brain. Its precise function is not well understood, but it is known to control or regulate the pituitary and adrenal glands. In ancient esoteric and spiritual systems, the pineal gland played a particularly important role: the seat of spiritual experience. In the Hindu understanding, the pineal gland represents the "third eye."

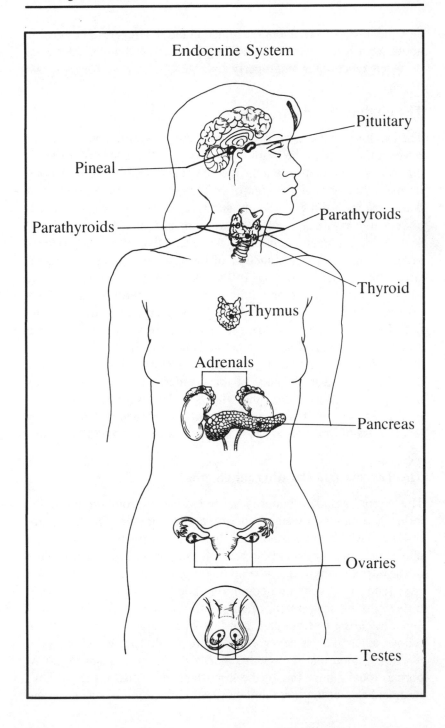

Endocrine System

Not enough is known about the pineal gland, however, to be specific about what it does when functioning properly and what it does not do when functioning improperly.

The Pituitary Gland

The pituitary gland is situated behind the bridge of your nose and beneath the floor of the brain. This tiny gland (the size of a pea) is the master gland controlling the rest of the endocrine system. Among its many functions is the control of those systems in the body that determine such things as height and rate of body development. An underactive pituitary produces dwarfism and retarded mental and sexual development in children. An overactive pituitary produces giantism. In women dysfunction of the pituitary disrupts the menstrual cycle. That's how the Pill works. It confuses the pituitary, fooling it into sending the wrong signals. The steroids that athletes take to produce extra muscle affect the pituitary. They decrease the flow of the hormone that triggers male testosterone. This in turn reduces the amount of sperm produced and also shrinks the testicles. The pituitary is particularly sensitive to sugar. Too much sugar disturbs the delicate balance of the pituitary, which in turn sends improper signals to all the other glands under its control. The result is a general rather than a specific malaise, affecting your energy level, sense of well-being, physical appearance, and overall identity.

The Thyroid and Parathyroid Glands

The thyroid gland, a butterfly-shaped organ in your throat, stores iodine and regulates weight, energy, and endurance. The four parathyroids (which are part of the thyroid) control the calcium and phosphorus metabolism of the body. If the thyroid secretes too much of the hormone thyroxine, the body's organs work at an accelerated pace, and this results in a condition called *hyperthyroidism*. If too little thyroxine is secreted, often due to a lack of iodine in the diet, *hypothyroidism* (weight gain and loss of energy) is a result. White refined sugar has an adverse effect on the thyroid gland. In fact, it's my opinion that too much sugar is one of the causes of osteoporosis today, since one of the important functions of the parathyroid, and also of the adrenal glands, is to break down and assimilate calcium. You can take large amounts of calcium and you won't get much benefit from it without reducing your intake of sugar.

If your thyroid gland is sluggish, you may experience physical and mental sluggishness, problems losing weight, decreased body temperature, puffiness in the hands and face, and (rarely) goiter, an enlarged thyroid gland. When your thyroid is overactive, you may experience extreme nervousness, weight loss and/or difficulty gaining weight, rapid pulse, bulging eyes—and eventually heart failure as the body's systems overwork trying to handle all the accelerated organic functions.

Both hyperactivity and underactivity of the thyroid often stem from a deficiency of iodine and zinc. In my experience, emotional stress can have a powerful adverse effect on the thyroid. But both conditions respond to biochemical reprogramming. On my diet program you would concentrate on those foods rich in iodine and zinc, especially in the mineral-rich products of the sea—dulse, kelp, even canned sardines. Six to ten shelled pumpkin seeds daily provide enough zinc to maintain normal thyroid function.

An underactive parathyroid gland does not process calcium and phosphorus efficiently, and mineral deposits build up in the arteries, setting you up for a heart attack or stroke. The solution is not increasing intake of calcium (either as dairy products or calcium supplements), since the gland will not process it. The causes of the dysfunctioning parathyroid are complex: lack of exercise, lack of sunshine (vitamin D), generally bad digestion, and emotional tension. All of these problems must be addressed to get the parathyroid working properly, plus a dietary emphasis on mineral-rich sea-derived foods. There is no quick fix.

The overactive parathyroid burns calcium up before it can be absorbed and even takes it away from the bones. This is osteoporosis, (brittle bones, bone deformities, bone cavities, and spontaneous fractures may occur). The overactive parathyroid responds to the same kind of treatment as the underactive parathyroid.

The Thymus Gland

The thymus is a cylindrical-shaped gland at the upper part of the breastbone, or sternum. The thymus masterminds the immune system. Under its control are the spleen, lymph nodes, bone marrow, tonsils, adenoids, appendix, and portions of the intestine. Until recently the thymus was regarded as an evolutionary leftover— useless, unproductive, and possibly even a source of trouble. Times change, however, and the thymus gland is now a hot item in medical research, the possible key to many health problems ranging from allergies and arthritis to cancer and aging. The thymus instructs certain white blood cells, called T-cells, what to attack and when. These T-cells in turn control other white blood cells that make antibodies. When the thymus gland no longer works efficiently, bacteria, viruses, and cancer cells are not attacked but are left free to attack the body themselves.

"The Thymus Thumper"

The thymus is the mastermind of the immune system, which today is under attack on all fronts. The Thymus thumper should be integrated into your exercise routine, right after skin brushing in the morning and whenever you can fit it in later in the day.

Make a fist. With the flat of your fist, give yourself a firm double thump on the top of the chest, about an inch below the hollow of the throat. Don't hit so hard that it hurts. Repeat 30 times to the rhythm of a heartbeat.

The Adrenal Glands

Two little cap-shaped glands on top of each kidney are the crucial adrenals. They secrete a substance called *adrenaline*, which determines your level of energy and endurance. The adrenals also regulate blood pressure; salt, protein, carbohydrate, mineral, and pigment metabolism; and, with the parathyroids, calcium metabolism. The adrenal glands are extremely sensitive to sugar. Foods such as chocolate, cola, and coffee have an adverse effect on these sensitive glands. Why? The caffeine and theobromine overstimulate and gradually weaken the adrenals, ending in malfunction. The adrenals manufacture cortisone, which regulates calcium metabolism—the way you assimilate and absorb calcium.

The painful joints of arthritics are often the result of massive deposits of calcium. Recognizing the role of cortisone in calcium assimilation, the medical profession often prescribes an animal-derived course of cortisone. Though this relieves the pain temporarily, the long-term effects are often catastrophic. The secret is not to have calcium build up in the first place, but if it occurs, to treat it nutritionally, gradually decreasing dependency on painkillers and palliatives.

What happens when your adrenals are underactive or overactive? Underactive adrenal glands tend to produce low blood pressure, particularly in women. They also are now generally acknowledged as a prime factor in skin, respiratory (asthma), and digestive allergies. If not too far deteriorated, the adrenals respond swiftly to proper nutrition. Overactive adrenals tend to produce high blood pressure, more so in men. Doctors often prescribe a diuretic, but this overworks the delicate kidneys, eventually ending up in dysfunction. Moreover, the patient becomes totally dependent upon the drug, which as in so many instances addresses only the symptom, not the cause. Proper nutrition brings the adrenals swiftly back into line.

The Pancreas and Islets of Langerhans

The pancreas is about six inches long, weighs about three ounces, and is located in front of the spine, below the stomach. The pancreas produces enzymes that digest food and convert it into assimilable nutrients. The islets of Langerhans (which are part of the pancreas) produce insulin, which controls the balance of sugar in the body.

What happens when the pancreas and islets of Langerhans work improperly? When the pancreas cannot do its job, food is not properly digested and, in effect, you suffer from malnutrition no matter how much food you're eating. Like most of the other glands, the pancreas is extremely sensitive to sugars and overrich and overrefined foods of all sorts. A diseased pancreas and sluggish liver amount to a kind of malnutrition of the overprivileged. Given half a chance and depending upon age, the pancreas responds swiftly to good treatment.

If the pancreas produces too much insulin, the result is low blood sugar, or hypoglycemia. The insulin is burning the glucose out of the blood, not leaving enough in the blood for metabolic purposes. How would you know? You may experience dizziness, nausea, anxiety, a feeling of faintness, and in extreme cases, convulsions and coma. Since glucose is the primary food for the brain, as well as for all the other cells in the body, the nervous systems are particularly vulnerable once hypoglycemia sets in.

If the pancreas secretes too little insulin, the body cannot process carbohydrates into a usable form, resulting in diabetes. Symptoms are insatiable thirst, fatigue, weakness, and emaciation. If diabetic patients have not been taking large insulin doses over a long period of time, they will respond to nutrition therapy; otherwise, the damage is largely irreversible.

The Ovaries and the Testes

The ovaries and the testes are the reproductive glands. The ovaries produce the seed (ovum) in women; the testes produce the sperm cells in men. The male hormone *testosterone* is responsible for the male sex drive, and the continued efficient production of testosterone is effectively the male fountain of youth. In women, the reproductive glands not only control the physical reproductive system but are also intimately connected to emotional and psychological states. As with all other glands, the ovaries and testes are highly sensitive and react adversely to improper diet: In men the sperm count can drop dramatically, and in both sexes the sex drive is seriously slowed down.

A diet rich in vitamin E, best attained from whole grains, especially millet and brown rice, and also avocados, often gradually regenerates the reproductive system.

The Lymphatic System

The lymphatic system is sometimes called the sewage system of the body. Its principal role is the removal of waste in the form of undigested protein and dead tissue. The lymphatic system consists of a complex network of vessels that follow the vascular system, rather in the way that sewers and drainage ditches run along streets and highways. Through these vessels flows the lymph, a colorless, odorless liquid similar in composition to seawater. The lymphatic system is also a major food transporter, receiving nutrients from the blood and carrying them to areas the blood does not reach directly. The lymphatic system is home to the white blood cells and, therefore, instrumental in all bodily functions related to immunity and defense against disease or infection.

What happens when the lymphatic system doesn't drain properly? When the body is overloaded with waste, the system reacts like an overflowing sewer. The waste material cannot pass through the lymph nodes, which may be thought of as the connections or joints of the lymphatic system. The nodes become overloaded with toxins and form soft painful swellings, usually at the armpits, ankles, groin, and throat. Skin brushing along with diet is a very effective way of regenerating an ailing lymphatic system. Brushing breaks the viscous material into more fluid form, allowing the lymphatic system to process it as it should. This is one of the chief ways in which brushing defeats cellulite.

Directly or indirectly, brushing connects all the body's systems. Since each organ and the glandular system have anywhere from six to eight acupuncture points scattered over your body, you are certain to activate them when brushing even if you should accidentally miss a meridian or nerve connection. Many of my patients remark that brushing feels almost like having a chiropractic adjustment. This is no surprise, given all those connections. By stimulating all the body's systems and helping them work together, brushing leads directly to better health and helps prepare the way to the next important prong in my program: exercise.

CHAPTER 4

Exercise

"I was going along doing the program, and everything was fine until the progression seemed to level off. Dr. Jack patted me on the back and said, 'The missing link is exercise. You need exercise to help the digestive process.' I've been walking forty minutes a day for the past five years, and it really works."
—Mariann M.

Exercise is as essential to vigorous physical strength and health as breath is to life. Muscles weaken and will eventually degenerate if insufficiently exercised. But it's not only the external muscles that are affected. Most people don't realize that internal, involuntary muscles also need exercise. Without it, all the vital organs suffer: the liver becomes sluggish owing to poor circulation; the intestines and colon suffer because of slower peristalsis; bowel action slows down, with constipation the result; the heart goes flabby through inaction. The functions of life are eventually reduced. When the voluntary muscles—those muscles that we control—are allowed to languish, those that we don't control are not fully utilized, and they atrophy. When those we control are exercised, increased demands on the respiratory, digestive, and circulatory systems stimulate and strengthen the unseen muscles of the body, producing the proper conditions for normal and healthy tissue repair.

Exercise is the essential third prong of my three-prong Biochemical Reprogramming System. Again, let me stress that any one of the three will help you. If you just change your diet, you'll benefit. If you just brush, you will benefit. If you just exercise, you will benefit. But for total health, the three must be done in conjunction on a regular basis.

The heart is not the only muscle to pump blood. Exercise provides the heart with a fantastic support system. Every muscle is an auxiliary heart helping to pump blood. When a muscle contracts it squeezes blood toward the heart. When it relaxes it allows the muscle to be filled with blood, exactly like the heart. Healthy, strong muscles take the burden off the heart. Strong muscles, strong heart; weak muscles, weak heart. The heart was not made to work by itself.

We live in a sedentary society. The majority of Americans, both male and female, sit on their way to and from work, sit at work, and then sit in front of a TV or at a movie or in a restaurant. They are engaging in only a minimum amount of activity every twenty-four hours.

Compared with the endurance and stamina of many long-lived, so-called primitive, third world peoples, that of "civilized" people is minimal. In natural surroundings self-induced exercise is unnecessary. Hunting, digging, farming, running, climbing trees, carrying things—all are part of daily existence. Indians of the Amazon or the Bushmen of the Kalahari would look upon deliberate exercise as a form of madness. For them, life itself is exercise. For us, the matter is precisely contrary. Practically nobody in the space age engages in the kind of physical activity that could be called "exercise" in the normal course of the day. So we must impose exercise upon ourselves if we want to live in health. I recall a segment on "60 Minutes" several years ago on the subject of longevity. It started off with a man who appeared to be in his fifties, and on the voice-over Morley Safer said, "Here's Temoterbah. He's galloping through the woods at great speed, and he's ninety-eight years old. And he's on his way to his mother's birthday party." At the end of the segment, the mother, who is 132 years old, is *dancing* with her sons, who are 98 and 94. Will you be doing that? Will I?

Everybody, almost without exception, finishes school with the wrong idea about exercise and its importance. So-called physical education is not education at all. It is a system designed to spot the athletes who will play on the school teams and bring it prestige and glory. The other 98 percent of students are left to fend for themselves. No one teaches them—us!—the importance of long-term consistent physical fitness. Mass juvenile unfitness and obesity have become matters of grave national concern. A study of elementary school children in Michigan showed that the seeds of future sickness had already been sown. Forty-one percent had high cholesterol; 28 percent had high blood pressure; and almost all—98 percent— showed at least one major risk factor for heart disease.

Symptoms of Old Age

According to recent studies of adults, physiologists have found significant evidence that many of the classic symptoms of old age are the direct result of inactivity. The average person does less and less exercise as he or she gets older, and what we think of as symptoms of old age—shaking hands, tottering gait, and stiff joints—often stem from lack of exercise. The case against inaction has been brought by a wide array of medical authorities, many of whom may disagree violently on many other matters. But about lack of exercise, all agree. An adult who "suddenly" reaches middle age without constantly working to keep up his or her health and physical condition has quite a few unpleasant physical surprises in store. Here's what it leads to:

- Noticeable loss of muscle mass, muscle tone, and muscle strength
- Accumulation of fat that goes on easily but becomes more and more difficult to take off
- Reduction of motor ability, balance, flexibility, and reflex or reaction time
- Reduction in work capacity
- Increase in injuries such as dislocations, sprains, and strains in various body joints, especially knees, shoulders, and spine

* Increase in cholesterol and blood pressure levels
* Slower metabolism
* Decrease in suppleness and resilience of arteries
* Brittle bones (osteoporosis)
* Lack of harmony and coordination in the nine systems of the body (nervous system, digestive system, etc.)

Everybody gets older every day, but old age is a state of mind often conditioned by the state of the body. Do something about the state of your body, and you'll never get "old." Patients often come to me thinking they have arthritis or rheumatism, and in many instances they've been sitting on their butts for so long, their muscles have atrophied and their joints have stiffened. Getting them moving is not so easy sometimes, but in case after case, people who once hobbled into my office (some on crutches or with canes!) waltz in after a few months of conscientious exercise. And that includes a few who adamantly refused to change their dietary ways. Exercise is as important as that.

Everything—your heart, lungs, stomach, veins, and arteries —improves through exercise. This doesn't mean you have to run ten miles a day. In the last couple of years the returns have come in on exercise to the point of excess. The orthopedists', podiatrists', and chiropractors' offices are filled with disabled jogging fanatics who have pushed their bodies beyond nature's intentions, and there is now solid research on the dangers of overexercise. Too much exercise can be dangerous, even lethal. But you do have a choice. No matter what your age or state of health, there is usually some healthful type of exercise available to you.

It has been found that exercise should be moderate, varied, and paced. You need twenty minutes of vigorous exercise three times a week on alternate days to produce a positive effect on the heart and cardiovascular system. Not only should you practice different forms of moderate exercise, but you actually gain more if you give yourself rest days in between. This applies particularly to the more strenuous kinds of exercise, such as Nautilus and weights. This paced exercise prevents the body from adapting and keeps it in a constant building mode. In other words, you can actually work out less and get greater results.

STRETCHING

How to Begin Exercising When You've
Never Exercised Before

Most people don't think of stretching as exercise. And most people don't stretch. But stretching is very important, an extremely beneficial and rather pleasant kind of exercise. It is also essential to stretch out three to five minutes before starting any more strenuous form of exercise.

Stretching elongates the muscles, makes them resilient, and keeps joints limber. It is particularly important for maintaining normal spinal function. Regular stretching keeps you from shrinking as you get older. (Not everybody realizes that after forty the body tends to shrink.) As age increases, resilience, limberness, and endurance become more important than strength and speed. Moreover, the limber body you have developed by stretching will be much less prone to injury in those other forms of exercise that work the lungs and heart. Cats keep in shape almost entirely by stretching.

There is no one stretching exercise that is best for everyone. In my practice, I tend to prescribe stretching exercises on an individual basis. There are many good exercise books and videotapes providing detailed information on a variety of methods. I personally like "Exercise" by Herbert M. Shelton (Natural Hygiene Society, P. O. Box 2132, Huntington, CT 06483).

Remember, do not try to stretch suddenly when you are cold. Always begin your stretching sessions gradually, especially when it's cold. Stretching can tear muscles if you go at it with more enthusiasm than wisdom. You might want to run slowly in place for a few minutes to warm up.

When to Stretch

The nice thing about stretching is that you can do it at odd spots throughout the day as well as at scheduled times. Try to get in a few minutes of stretching early in the morning, after your skin brushing. Beyond that, look for opportunities during the day: at your desk, while watching television, while waiting for a pot to boil. Break long automobile rides with periodic short stretching sessions. If you look for places to stretch, you'll find them.

THE BREATH OF LIFE

Breathing is something we all take for granted. You can be eating the best organically grown food in the world in correct combinations, but if your breathing is shallow and constricted, you're not utilizing all that good food properly and you're not getting full benefit from it.

Here's a rough-and-ready way to judge your own breathing efficiency. Pay attention to the way you breathe. If your abdomen and stomach area is expanding noticeably with every inhalation, it means you are breathing deeply and more or less correctly. If your stomach and abdomen do not enter into the breathing process, your breathing is shallow. You are only using the top third of your lungs, and you need breathing exercises to get you breathing correctly. If on inhaling your stomach and diaphragm actually contract, your breathing is both incorrect and self-defeating. Another signal of improper breathing is if you find yourself involuntarily sighing or taking an extra breath in order to get air into your lungs.

Poor breathing is usually linked to poor posture. When you're not standing straight, your lungs cannot fill up properly. Exercise will improve both posture and the accessory breathing muscles. Better breathing will then become automatic. If you find that you are not breathing properly, then exercise regularly. Even if you are breathing properly, you will still benefit from specific breathing exercises.

I generally prescribe two separate but complementary kinds of breathing exercises. The first is mainly concerned with correct breathing technique and correct posture. The second is aimed at cleansing: at coaxing the lungs into getting rid of their accumulations of contaminants, toxins, and waste matter built up over years of city living, sedentary habits, and improper diet.

NOTE: Normally you breathe in through the nose and out through the nose. You'll notice when you first wake up in the morning, this is how you're breathing. But during exercise you want to get into the habit of breathing in through the nose and out through the *mouth*. This is actually the most natural form of breathing. If while doing your breathing exercises you start feeling light-headed (hyperventilation), rest briefly, then resume exercise slowly. Always do the breathing exercises with the window open or outdoors if possible. Here are a few of the most important:

1. Lying flat on your back, place a small pillow or a small rolled towel between your shoulder blades. Do not place a pillow under your head. Keep knees bent. Lift arms slowly up and backward overhead while you inhale through your nose for a slow count of 5. Slowly lower arms to sides while you exhale forcibly through your mouth for a count of 5. Exhale completely.

2. Seated on a firm chair, place hands behind your head with fingertips touching each other. Inhale deeply through your nose while pulling your flexed elbows backward and raising your chest, to a slow count of 5. Exhale forcibly through your open mouth to a slow count of 5. Exhale completely.

3. Seated on a firm chair, *quickly* inhale and exhale 10 times, then on the eleventh count, slowly inhale for 7 seconds, hold for 7 seconds, exhale for 7 seconds. Repeat whole procedure 3 times. Increase the time you hold your breath on the eleventh count 1 second per day until you are holding it for 14 seconds, then repeat the cycle, starting at 7 seconds.

4. Seated on a firm chair, inhale *slowly* through the nose. When lungs have been completely filled, exhale immediately with the lips pressed close to the teeth while keeping a narrow slit open between them. Through this narrow slit force the air out in a number of short, detached breaths. You should feel as though the mouth is not open at all, and that a great effort on the part of the abdominal, diaphragm, and rib muscles is required to force the air through the small opening. Repeat procedure 4 times.

5. As often as possible during the day, especially when in the open or when walking, fill your lungs to the fullest extent as many times as possible. A correct full breath should be taken in the following manner: Draw in all the breath you can through the nose, allowing the expansion to commence in the abdominal region, and gradually ascend to the chest. After you have drawn in all the breath you can, hold it for a moment and try to inhale another breath, and following this, exhale fully through the mouth. Repeat this exercise until a slight feeling of fatigue ensues.

EXERCISE

Now that you've done your stretching and breathing, you're ready to begin exercising. But before you begin, get a thorough physical checkup from your family physician—especially if you've never exercised before or not in years. You could have hidden problems that only a checkup would reveal.

Start Gently and Work Up Your Heartbeat

For all its therapeutic value, stretching will not get your heart and lungs working hard enough. For that you need something more strenuous. But don't worry. This doesn't mean you have to jump up and down with Jane Fonda. Aerobics can be any exercise that gets the lungs, heart, and vascular system working hard. Even walking can be aerobic if it's done fast enough. Though you may not believe it, moderate exercise gradually undertaken gives the quickest results.

I have seen winter-heavy patients get summer-slim in a matter of weeks on a regime of moderate exercise, brushing, and diet. NOTE: If something hurts, stop doing it. Things to watch out for: problems recovering your wind once you're out of breath; light-headedness; racing heartbeat that does not quickly recover once you stop; trouble sleeping at night and/or nausea following exercise (a sign of overexertion). After exercise you should feel good, but tired. If all you feel is tired, chances are you are overexerting.

The Secret Is Regularity and Enjoyment

There are many viable and valuable exercises to choose from. The trick is to find one you really enjoy. It's essential that you stimulate your heart, but that can be agony if your heart's not in it. Jogging may be a natural for lean loners who enjoy the challenge and the solitude but sheer torture for those whose frames and whose personalities are not suited to it. Find an exercise or, better yet, a couple of exercises that you like and that present a perpetual challenge. The more "intelligent" the exercise, the less liable you are to get bored with it. Without pretending to provide an all-inclusive list, here are the exercises I tend to recommend and the reasons I recommend them.

Walking

Walking is something I recommend to everyone, except those with special problems like gouty and heavily arthritic patients or those with knee and spinal problems or those with phlebitis. Everyone can walk. It's the first thing we learn after crawling. Most of us like to walk. And walking is one of the easiest and best fat-busters and inch-shrinkers. Walking briskly (dawdling is useless) gets your heart pumping, your lungs working, and just about all the muscles and joints of your body exercised. It gives the same benefit as jogging and causes less wear and tear on the body. You'll find very few walkers in the waiting rooms of the podiatrists and orthopedists. At sixty or even seventy you can still walk with great vigor. Walking is by far the best exercise for those who have had coronary problems of one kind or another, but it's absolutely essential to consult a physician before embarking on a program. Coronary sufferers can definitely improve the cardiovascular function through regular walking. A British Medical Association survey found almost no heart or weight problems in regular walkers. Research has shown that walking begun early in life slows the aging process.

Another advantage to walking is that it's free, or almost. All you need is a good stout pair of comfortable shoes and the space to walk in. Initially it would appear that walking is almost immune to commercialization, but I notice that Yankee ingenuity has even found a way around this. There are walking fashions, walking magazines, special walking shoes, walking socks, walking weights, and Walkmans. I've not seen anyone yet advertising a special walking dog, but a dog provides one of the best of all possible excuses for acquiring a walking habit. You may think of a thousand good reasons not to go for a walk on any given day, but your dog will not accept any of them. Whatever it takes to get you walking, buy in.

Since we all know how to walk, advice on the subject may sound superfluous. But there is a right way and a wrong way to walk, just as there is a right way and wrong way to breathe and eat. In natural surroundings we would be walking barefoot on the earth, sand, grass, or other resilient surface, and no one would have to pay attention to walking technique. But on concrete or asphalt improper walking can jolt and jar your frame and create skeletal problems.

Mainly you want to remember not to put all your weight down hard on the heel. The outer part of the heel should hit the ground first and you roll along the outside of the foot and step off the ball of the foot, pushing with your toes. Be conscious of the role played by your toes. Usually, with our feet encased in shoes, we pay no attention to the toes. Once you become aware of them, you'll see how important they are to correct walking. What you're after is an easy rolling gait. Your arms swing free, your posture is erect, you don't look at the ground. You'll find your breathing takes care of itself as you find your proper pace.

Walk briskly. Start with a half a mile to a mile. Gradually increase both pace and distance until you're striding out covering a mile in fifteen to twenty minutes. (Four miles an hour is the army pace.) Six miles a day is the ideal, but in practice this is not so easily achieved. Aim for an hour a day and your body will thank you for the rest of your life.

Swimming: A Great Exercise
for Those who Hate to Exercise

Are you one of the many people who avoid exercise but wish you could increase your energy, improve your posture, and lose a few pounds? Swimming, says the National Swimming Institute, is the exercise for those who hate exercise. It's a fact that many people who hate getting into a sweat in a gym do not mind putting the same amount of energy into laps in a pool. Recognized by coaches and trainers in all sports as the best all-around physical conditioner and as an exercise for all age groups, swimming is rapidly growing more popular.

No other physical activity provides so much exercise without the risks inherent in body-contact sports or the bone, joint, and muscle (musculoskeletal) problems that plague tennis and handball players, gymnasts, runners, weight lifters, and other noncontact sports players.

The benefits of consistent daily swimming are directly proportional to age. Most physical problems in the over-fifty age group are heart- or weight-related. Both may be helped or overcome by regular swimming.

Swimming is less likely than any other sport to cause a sudden shock to the heart, since a swimmer's pulse rate usually increases gradually, not abruptly. The buoyancy of the water also allows exercise of many muscles that are rarely if ever used in the normal dry world.

Flexibility

For the elderly, flexibility is more important than mere strength and endurance. Another blessing of water exercise is that it rarely if ever causes aching muscles. In addition to improving your physical appearance and condition, there is considerable evidence that swimming has a sedative effect on the nervous system. The swimmer finishes mentally and emotionally relaxed. (Regular, systematic walking has a similar effect.) Swimming is being used increasingly in psychotherapy for the treatment of emotional tension.

Aerobics

Aerobics, as I've said, is a name applied to any exercise whose main focus is to get lungs, heart, and vascular system working hard. Running, walking, swimming, bicycling, rowing, and sports that require constant action are all aerobic exercises. Basketball and dancing are aerobic; bowling and golf are not aerobic.

Specific aerobic exercise classes are not essential. But for many people the combination of discipline and camaraderie of the aerobics class provides the inspiration to overcome the bodily inertia that is the lot of most of us. Whatever it takes to get you working your lungs, heart, and vascular system hard is the aerobic exercise for you. I do find among my patients, however, that specific aerobics classes are generally more suitable for the young. There is a tendency among older people to overdo it, with actual physical problems as a result. As always, moderation is the key.

Rowing

I find the rowing machine a terrific exercise. It exercises just about every muscle in the body. It's aerobic, too. Injuries are almost unheard-of, and rain, snow, or heat waves will not give you the excuse to avoid it. Your little rowing machine fits handily in the corner of a room. Ten to twenty minutes a day (or at least three or four times a week), and your body gets fit and stays young. Rowing is a splendid maintenance exercise, particularly as you get older. It really stops you from going downhill. I use my rowing machine three times a week.

Bicycling

Bicycling is a fine exercise. To be out there in the fresh air, pedaling away, watching the miles and the scenery slip by, is a fine way to coerce the body into an aerobic frame of mind. Or it would be were it not for another even more ingenious invention, the automobile. To my mind, bicycling on empty country roads counts as one of the great pleasures of life. But bicycling anywhere else seems to me so consistently hazardous as to outweigh whatever pleasures and advantages a bicycle otherwise possesses. Stationary bicycles, on the other hand, pose no risks. I think it just depends upon how important it is to you to see the scenery slipping by.

Jumping Rope

This is good exercise for people in a hurry. Jumping rope gets your heart and lungs working harder in less time than almost anything else. The equipment is dead cheap. The space needed to practice is minimal, and experienced jumpers get into a rhythm that becomes intensely pleasurable, despite the hard work. There is only one drawback to jumping rope. People with spinal problems should approach it cautiously and always jump with both feet.

The Martial Arts

The Eastern disciplines alone among physical activities provide the opportunity for constant growth, lifelong learning. They contain the spiritual element that plays a part in everyday life—a "genius" element that no purely physical Western exercise can touch. The purely physical exercises work the body but not the emotions, the soul, or the mind. The difference between the Eastern forms of exercise and others is roughly the difference between practicing scales and playing a violin.

Many people have the wrong idea about the martial arts. The martial arts should not be equated with Kung Fu movies or *The Karate Kid*. The "hard" contact martial arts—karate, tae kwon do, judo—are rough, dangerous, competitive. Those no longer young and fit should seriously consider the risks. On the other hand, those in their fifties and even sixties can embark upon the "soft" martial arts—aikido, tai chi chuan—with impunity. Actually, as long as you can walk you are never too old for tai chi chuan. The martial arts are hard work, but for those who enjoy the challenge they are a brilliant means for getting and staying fit.

Yoga

Many of my patients who can't do regular exercises thrive on yoga. This does not mean yoga should be considered a last resort for the semi-invalid. The benefit of yoga is that it provides the same kind of inner and outer exercise as the martial arts but without the fighting basis. There are many forms of yoga. The yoga associated with physical disciplines is called hatha-yoga. This involves asanas, or postures, specifically developed over thousands of years, designed to exercise body, mind, and soul simultaneously.

Yoga can be practiced at every level of intensity, from the gentlest to the most demanding. Yoga stretches and exercises virtually every muscle in the body, including many untouched by other forms of exercise. Yoga massages the internal organs and enhances the circulation of blood throughout the body. It cleanses and helps balance the endocrine system.

Yoga is best studied under a master, but with good books and video readily available, can be practiced alone. It is odd that the very best exercises seem to require the least paraphernalia. All you need for yoga is yourself and a quiet place to sit or lie down.

EXERCISE TIPS

• Never exercise on a full stomach. Always exercise on an empty stomach, at least two to three hours after a meal.
• You will lose large quantities of body fluids if you exercise strenuously, particularly on hot, humid days. Drink plenty of water during and after your sessions to offset dehydration. It's dehydration that accounts for that tired feeling.
• Walk without shoes whenever convenient. The pores of your feet need to breathe without restriction. Shoes invariably restrict your feet, and today most shoes are partially or wholly synthetic, further complicating the problem.
NOTE: Those with neuro-circulatory ailments such as phlebitis or neuropathy should not walk barefoot.
• Consistency, along with moderation, is the key to successful exercise.
• Make sure you know the difference between pain and exertion.
• Exercise is supposed to be pleasurable work, not torture.
• Remember, exercise is not optional if health is your goal.

Exercise Gimmicks

There's a devil in the flesh, and he is a lazy devil. Sometimes we have to be smarter than he is to get our bodies into action. So here are a few gimmicks accumulated over the years from my patients and various other sources:

• Put your sneakers next to your favorite chair to remind you of your program.
• Try an exercise cassette or record. Make it part of your exercise program to turn it on as soon as you come home from work.

• When watching TV, don't just sit there. Do ten leg-lifts or toe-touches while in your chair. Get up and stretch during the commercial breaks.

• Stand up while you talk on the phone. Use the time to tighten thigh and buttock muscles.

• Turn on the radio and clean the house to some peppy music.

• Walk to work if you can, or park your car far enough away to force a walk.

• When in a car or plane, sitting or standing, get your toes moving. It helps pump the heart. So whenever you're stationary for long periods of time, wiggle your toes.

• Write a "fitness contract" for yourself. "I will walk, run, or bike every day for a month." Sign it and check off each day as you follow the program.

• Make exercise a game. Look for reasons to put little exercise episodes into your day. Every set of stairs should be a challenge. I winter in an apartment in Florida, and I make a point of running the five flights, two steps at a time.

Physician, Heal Thyself

Well into my seventies, I still walk four brisk miles a day almost without fail. I also work out with dumbbells, on a rowing machine, and on a stationary bicycle. I swim all year around. I also work out on a speed punching bag, which not only is terrific for aerobics but is an upper arm toner and sharpens hand-eye coordination.

CHAPTER 5

Three Natural Healing Diets

By now you know I believe your body was not designed to be constantly abused and that it will eventually break down through daily maltreatment and faulty nutrition. To undo the damage, I have designed three diets to induce cleansing, detoxification, and healing of the body. Moreover, on each diet you will lose weight (although even the Weight-Loss Diet is primarily a cleansing diet) and you will notice a higher energy level and a feeling of well-being.

Note: I use the word "diet" because no better word comes readily to mind. But what I really mean is a way of integrating the foods you eat into your lifestyle in such a way that you get healthy and stay healthy without turning yourself into a fanatic or social pariah. I want to warn you, however, that problems may arise. Think of this detoxification period as similar to spring cleaning. Your house is in turmoil. So if you feel some discomfort, take heart. It means the diet is working. Spring cleaning has begun.

Each diet allows for eating what you want and inevitable lapses. Never again will you have to count a single calorie or weigh portions of food. You can eat as much as you want until satisfied. At no time will you get that "restricted diet" feeling—a common complaint of diet followers.

You may find it easier to start off with a fruit breakfast and your usual lunch and dinner. In a week or so, eat fruit for breakfast and a Dr. Jack lunch. When you have adjusted to this, you will be ready to phase into dinners. (People seem to have the most trouble with their dinners.)

The Three Natural Healing Diets follow in this order: (1) Long Life Diet, (2) Supreme Diet, and (3) Weight-Loss Diet. Each diet in combination with the dry brushing and exercise will maintain the body in perfect condition. The Three Natural Healing Diets are based upon the acid/alkaline principle, the principles of food combining, and my rules for intelligent eating.

To get the most out of these diets, observe the following:

ACID/ALKALINE PRINCIPLE

To preserve the normal alkalinity of your body, which I described at length in chapter 2, you should eat 60 to 70 percent health-promoting "alkaline foods"—fresh fruits and vegetables rich in organic minerals and vitamins, especially when you also eat acid-forming foods (you know which they are!). There is no reason to exclude acid-forming foods, and if you use them judiciously and in correct balance, they will do no harm and in fact will be beneficial.

Since the healthy body must have mostly *living* mineral and alkaline foods, it is best to eat fruits at breakfast (although I have alternated fruit breakfasts with grain breakfasts to make the transition easier). For lunch, eat fresh fruit or vegetable salads, soups, or vegetable sandwiches. At dinner, eat vegetables, especially fresh salads, and occasional animal protein. Eat cereal products sparingly—no more than I indicate.

To be sure you stay well, plan your meals to follow the valuable acid/alkaline chart on pages 23–24. Don't become fanatical. Just be reasonable. You can indulge in an all-acid-forming meal, but make sure your next two or three meals are predominantly alkaline-forming foods.

PRINCIPLES OF FOOD COMBINING

When I started in practice, only a few health advocates were stressing scientific food combining, which simply means the combining of certain foods for more efficient digestion. It takes considerable strength and energy for the body to utilize and digest food. Combining foods incorrectly throws a monkey wrench into the mechanics of digestion. The body is not designed to digest more than one concentrated (low water content) food at a time. Fruits are not concentrated. Vegetables are not concentrated. Grains and animal proteins *are* concentrated.

Eating poorly combined foods forces your digestive system to perform several conflicting tasks simultaneously. Digesting acid-inducing foods calls for quite different action from digesting alkaline-inducing foods. When foods are improperly combined, they stay in the digestive tract much longer than they should, creating toxins and wasting energy.

Here are the chief rules of food combining (NOTE: See chart p. 23):

1. *Always eat fruit on an empty stomach.* Fruits are easily digestible. If you eat them with any other food (especially vegetables and grains), the other food combines with the fruit and prevents the body from absorbing nutrients quickly and swiftly eliminating the waste. All fruits, except for bananas, dates, and dried fruit, stay in the stomach an hour or two. If you eat a fruit with a grain or vegetable, it stays in the stomach much longer (three hours or more) and forms acids instead of alkalines, so you are not getting the full benefit of the fruit.

2. *Vegetables combine with almost everything.* Vegetables combine with everything except fruit. There are starchy and non-starchy vegetables. Starchy vegetables should not be eaten with a protein. Since cooking carrots, for example, transforms them from a nonstarchy to a starchy vegetable, they should not be eaten with a protein meal, although raw carrots would be okay. See chart on page 23 for detailed information.

3. *Never eat sweet foods with meals.* Never combine sugars or sweets with anything else. Yes, this means no desserts. Sugars combined with other foods ferment in the digestive system and form toxins and gas. As everyone knows, when you eat pancakes with syrup for breakfast you taste them all day long. Now you know why. When I have my own ice cream fix, I have it between meals. When you have a sweet tooth, try satisfying it with sweet, juicy fruit.

4. *Starches are the easiest combinations.* Eat starch with another starch or with any vegetable. For example, a meal of brown rice with steamed carrots, corn bread, and butter would be fine. *Note:* Most people don't realize that all grains with the exception of millet (a protein grain) are starches and the same rules apply (see chart, page 23).

5. *Go easy on fats.* There is not much to say about fats and oils except that you should eat them as sparingly as possible. Remember, fats do not combine with protein. That means go easy on bacon and eggs and sautéed meats. With my food combining system you will get the fats your body needs naturally in an easy-to-assimilate form. Look at the menus on pages 105–117 to see how easy it is.

6. *And now for the proteins.* Eat protein with a vegetable, never with a starch. That's right. You never eat steak with potatoes. Why not? Animal proteins alone or in correct combination will go through your digestive system in four hours or so. Starch alone or in correct combination will go through your system in two to three hours. But combining protein and starch takes six to eight hours just to get out of the stomach, and that's too long. It is a sticky concentrated combination with little fiber content, and it takes too long to get through the small and large intestines. Toxins are created, acids are produced, and the acid/alkaline balance is upset.

NOTE: *Tomatoes are the golden food.* Many of my patients think they are allergic to tomatoes. In my opinion, ripe tomatoes are one of the best detoxifiers we have. If you break out after eating tomatoes, it is often because they are cleansing your body of toxins through the skin, the largest eliminative organ. So if you are sensitive, approach tomatoes carefully to avoid too strong a reaction. Tomatoes act as a catalyst and neutralize the harmful uric acid found in all animal proteins. So when you eat animal protein or dairy foods, try to eat tomatoes. Fresh vine-ripened tomatoes are the best.

In winter go for the cherry or plum tomatoes. In a pinch, canned tomatoes will do.

The food combining rules above provide a framework for your day-to-day eating. The food principles below are more like the Ten Commandments—specific do's and don'ts for permanent health.

FOOD PRINCIPLES

• *Eat only when hungry.* Do not eat except when hungry. This sounds obvious, but it isn't. Most of us eat out of habit and not out of hunger. The body doesn't need food when it's not hungry and therefore not as many enzymes are working to digest the food. The food turns to fat, and who wants more fat? Eating when not hungry is the main reason so many Americans are overweight. If your appetite is poor, you will find it increases when concentrated foods, such as sugar and meat, are restricted.

• *Eat juicy foods prior to concentrated foods.* I call "juicy" foods all those foods with a high water content. Salads and raw vegetables are juicy foods. Meats, grains, and dairy products are concentrated foods. You should eat your juicy foods first for psychological as well as dietary reasons. Most of us are hooked on meats and concentrated foods. But it is the vegetables that do us the most good. So if we eat our juicy foods first, we won't crave as much meat or other concentrated food. It's as simple as that.

• *Eat animal source foods in moderation.* If you must eat animal protein, never eat it more than once a day. And try not to eat it on consecutive days.

• *Eat small meals and only enough to satisfy your appetite.* Do not overeat. When you overeat at any one meal, you overload your digestive tract. Eat small meals five or six times a day if you have to, in order to satisfy your hunger. Hypoglycemics, take note: Frequent small meals spaced throughout the day tend to maintain your blood sugar level.

• *Do not drink liquids with meals.* Liquids dilute the enzymes necessary for digestion; if you follow my diets, you will get the water you need from the fruits and vegetables. You'll lose the craving for wine, beer, water, or soda to wash the food down. As a rule of thumb, no liquids an hour before eating or two hours after.

• *Chew foods to a near liquid state.* One of the very first and most important steps of digestion takes place in the mouth. If you don't chew thoroughly, you place an additional burden on the internal digestive organs. They must work harder to do their job. In time, through overwork, they break down. They do not secrete as many digestive enzymes as they once did, and the whole process suffers, causing indigestion, gas fermentation, and a host of other problems. So, chew!

• *Drink and cook with distilled water.* Distilled water is water that has been heated until it turns to steam and then cooled so that it condenses back to water. All impurities, minerals, and chemicals are removed in the process. You are getting actual 100 percent pure water. This will begin to clean out your arteries, your liver, your kidneys, etc. It acts as a solvent. (See page 224 for more on water.)

Large companies selling water softeners have cleverly campaigned against distilled water. Their claim is that distilled water is leaching the minerals out of your body. Exactly! These minerals were formerly lining your arteries, kidneys, bladder, liver, and gallbladder where they do not belong.

• *Do not drink or eat when in pain, upset, or overly tired.* Your body is so involved with the emotional state or with your pain that it does not produce the required amounts of digestive enzymes.

• *Eat dinner at least three hours before bedtime.* Normal bodily wear and tear is repaired at night during sleep. Your body cannot simultaneously digest food and carry out these repair functions effectively if you go to bed on a full stomach.

• *Always drink lemon juice in lukewarm or tepid water before bedtime.* Lemon juice is a tremendous alkalizer, neutralizer, and antiseptic—probably the best we have. Take it just before bedtime. Your dinner should be digested already, and the lemon juice can work its wonders unimpeded. Start with the juice of half a medium lemon in a half-glass of lukewarm or tepid water.

Work up to one lemon. For those who have sleeping problems, this is the greatest natural sedative. *Note:* Rinse your mouth out afterward with plain water or brush your teeth. Occasionally there is a reaction between the lemon juice and tooth enamel. Only use fresh-squeezed lemon. NOTE: Lemons are not indicated for those suffering from ulcers.

THE LONG LIFE DIET

The Long Life Diet is designed to take the stress off the digestive and metabolic systems. These systems are under attack from a number of fronts. Among them:

1. *SAD*—the Standard American Diet (see page 236–7). Briefly, here, let's just say that the Standard American Diet is appalling and something has to be done about it.
2. *Internal contaminants*—chemical additives, preservatives, and hormones have invaded and poisoned our food supplies.
3. *External contaminants*—the air we breathe and the water we drink are highly toxic and tainted, with so many pollutants the EPA cannot count them.
4. *Drugs and medication*—apart from the obvious dangers of narcotics, Americans in general overdose themselves with medication that does much harm and little good.
5. *The rat race*—life in later twentieth-century America is a rat race. Everyone knows this. Very few are unaffected.

In our modern environment we can never eliminate all these problems, but the Long Life Diet is designed to help us cope with them in good health and with good heart. Follow this diet and you will see the difference. Soon! Increased energy. Calmer nerves. Better digestion.

The Long Life Diet allows for five days on and two nonconsecutive days off, each week.

Days On

Breakfast will be fresh fruit or cereal. Lunch will be vegetable or fruit salads, soups, or sandwiches. Dinners are always a large salad and vegetables, grains, or occasionally pasta and animal protein.

Days Off: "Eat What You Want" Days

Your "eat what you want" days are any *two days* a week you choose. You can change them from week to week, but they should *never* be two consecutive days.

Of course, the closer you stick to the program, the sooner you will feel its benefits.

On "eat what you want" days you can indulge in "forbidden" food combinations: bacon and eggs for breakfast, fish and brown rice for dinner, or sweets for dessert.

You should realize, however, that the Long Life Diet cleanses and detoxifies your body. Because of "housecleaning," a day of excessive eating may take its toll. If so, realize you feel that way as a result of what you ate and not of this program.

Note: Even though it is an "eat what you want" day, if you want to do yourself a big nutritional favor, make lunch or dinner a fruit meal to help you neutralize the effects of improper eating. If you want to go out for Sunday brunch, fine, but try to adhere to the fruit meal later in the day.

Fruit Meals on "Eat What You Want" Days

The fruit meal for lunch or dinner on your "eat what you want" days should consist of up to *two types of fruits*.

• Acid fruit will be the most beneficial on your "eat what you want" days.*

---

*There is no easy way out of this confusion of terminology. The fruits that taste acid and contain a high percentage of acid are those that induce the body into producing alkalines. So you eat the acid fruits to redress the acid/alkaline imbalance of the body and to make the imbalance more alkaline.

- Sub-acid fruit will be second best.
- Sweet fruit will have no neutralizing effect.

On your "eat what you want" days, have the juice of *two* medium fresh squeezed lemons (depending on your tolerance) in a glass of warm water (you can add ½ teaspoon of raw, uncooked honey) before retiring.

Breakfast Notes

It is important that all your fruits be *fresh* and *ripe*.

Be *reasonable*—eat *seasonal*. Make substitutions for the following meals by choosing seasonal foods. (For example, when cherries are ripe and the price is right, eat cherries, and so on.)

Be sure your fruits are *properly combined*. If occasionally these recipes or your recipes are not in keeping with the food combining principles, it's okay. It's important that your lifestyle not be disrupted.

The breakfast recipes are all for one serving; eat as much as you need to satisfy your hunger, and no more.

Make a "Blender Beauty" for any breakfast. Mix two properly combined fruits with up to ½ cup of apple juice, 1 level tsp. of sesame tahini and/or 1 level tsp. of lecithin granules, and blend to desired consistency.

In winter include dried fruits such as raisins, currants, or figs in your menus to maintain your body warmth.

When preparing a fruit plate, be sure to arrange the fruit attractively for eye appeal. Japanese and other Eastern cultures understand the importance of aesthetics in cuisine.

Be creative and use your imagination. These are only suggestions. Pick the fruits and grains you enjoy best.

Purchase all nuts, seeds, grains, and dried fruit in your health food store or the health sections of progressive supermarkets.

Before purchasing apple juice for your cereals, read the labels. Buy unfiltered, unpasteurized juices that are not made from concentrate.

Butter: Use sweet stick butter for cooking and sweet whipped butter for spreading.

Appetite Suppressant

Add fresh coconut to your fruit meals. Eat as much as you want. It acts as an *appetite suppressant*. It's a bit of work, but well worth your efforts. It's delicious! Puncture one of the "eyes" on the coconut and pour off the milk. This milk, unpolluted and unadulterated, is filled with vitamins and minerals. Put the whole coconut in a preheated 450-degree oven for 4 to 5 minutes. Put it on a hard surface (preferably outside) and hit it with a hammer. The shell shatters and separates from the meat. Store the peeled coconut chunks in a jar in the refrigerator, covered with water.

Lunch and Dinner Notes

On mornings when you have cereals or grains, have fruit for lunch.
Remember: Be *reasonable*—eat *seasonal*. Make sure all your vegetables, particularly tomatoes, are ripe. When corn is in season, eat it two or three nights a week as your main dish (preferably raw or lightly steamed) with a salad, another vegetable, and whole-grain bread.
You can make any substitutions you'd like with your lettuce greens, using anything except iceberg. In the quest for crispness, most of the nutrition has been bred out of iceberg lettuce.
When buying carrots, keep in mind that California carrots are sweeter and more easily digested than Florida or Texas carrots—because of the different soil.

Salad Dressings

You can save time and effort by using prepared natural dressings sold in your health food store. Just read the labels and know what you're buying. You really don't need fancy salad dressings; a lot of my patients like to drizzle cold pressed oil and fresh-squeezed lemon juice over their salads, and they're happy. Here are some recipes in case you get bored:

¼ c. sesame (or other cold-pressed) oil
3 T. lemon juice
½ tsp. minced fresh dill

Mix ingredients well with a fork and pour over salad.

(Serves 2)

¼ c. extra virgin olive oil
Juice of ½ lemon
2 tsp. of any combination of fresh minced herbs of your
choice, such as oregano, parsley, basil, or dill, or ½ tsp.
dried

With a fork, mix ingredients well and pour over salad.

(Serves 2)

The next three healthy and delicious salad dressings are from
The Vegan Kitchen cookbook, by Freya Dininshah. *The Vegan Kitchen*
is available from the American Vegan Society, 501 Old Harding
Highway, Malaga, NJ 08328.

THE VEGAN AVOCADO DRESSING

½–1 avocado (depending on size)
½ c. tomato juice

Blend mashed avocado with tomato juice.

(Yields ¾–1 c.)

THE VEGAN TOMATO-PARSLEY DRESSING

1 large tomato
¼ c. soy oil
4 sprigs parsley

Buzz all ingredients in blender.

(Yields ¾ c.)

THE VEGAN VEGETABLE DRESSING

    1 stick celery
    ½ sweet bell pepper
    ½ cucumber
    4 sprigs parsley
    ¼ c. corn oil
    Juice of 1 lemon

Buzz all ingredients in blender.

(Yields ¾ c.)

VARIATIONS: If you don't have a particular ingredient the recipe calls for, be creative and substitute what's on hand.

Steaming Vegetables

Use a vegetable-steaming basket. Put the vegetables in the basket and place in a saucepan to which ¾ inch water has been added. (Of course, use more water to steam foods that have to cook longer, such as potatoes or beets.) Bring to the point of steaming, then lower heat to medium-low. Cook with lid on until vegetables are tender.

Oils

Use cold-pressed oils, such as safflower, sesame, black sesame, or olive oil. When using olive oil for cooking, use virgin; when using it in dishes such as salads, where it won't be cooked, use extra virgin olive oil. It's best to buy your oils in the health food store; keep them refrigerated to prevent them from going rancid.

Bread

It is also best to buy your breads in the health food store. Try different varieties, such as sourdough rye, corn, whole-grain, soy, etc. Whole wheat bread is not recommended (because of its high gluten content—many otherwise mysterious allergies can be traced to gluten) and should be kept to a minimum. Excellent breads are made by Essene and Shiloh Farms. You can also order bread from Walnut Acres. See the mail-order list in the back of the book for their address.

THE LONG LIFE DIET

FIRST WEEK—MONDAY

Breakfast

Fiesta Fruit Salad

Grapefruit, peeled, membrane removed, and chopped
Apple, peeled, cored, and chopped
Grapes
Shredded coconut

Mix as much grapefruit, apple, and grapes as you want. Garnish with coconut.

Lunch

Avocado Vegetable Bowl

Dinner

Sunny Spinach Salad
Baked potato with butter
Steamed broccoli with oil and lemon

Breakfast

Hawaiian Float

½ pineapple (cut lengthwise)
Strawberries, halved
Kiwi fruit, peeled and chopped
Bite-size chunks of fresh coconut

Remove pineapple from its rind and chop. Refill shell with chopped pineapple, strawberries, kiwi, and coconut.

Lunch

The Great Mohican, with cucumber or carrot sticks

Dinner

Red Leaf Avocado Salad
Pasta à la Richard, or
Chicken Oreganato with tomatoes
Steamed asparagus

FIRST WEEK—WEDNESDAY

Breakfast

Grain Morning: granola, puffed millet, millet flakes, or puffed corn
   mixed with apple juice

Lunch

Fruit Delight

Dinner

Plaza Salad
Vegetable Stir-fry
Brown rice

FIRST WEEK—THURSDAY

Breakfast

Blender Beauty

> 2 peaches, peeled and chopped
> 1 banana, peeled and chopped
> ½ c. blueberries
> ⅓ c. yogurt
> ⅛–¼ c. apple juice (optional)
> 1 tsp. lecithin granules
>
> Combine all ingredients in a blender and mix thoroughly.

Lunch

Carrot Waldorf Salad

Dinner

Carrot juice
Dr. Jack's Garden Salad
Susan's Creamy Potato-Cabbage Soup
Southern style Corn bread

FIRST WEEK—FRIDAY

Breakfast

EAT WHAT YOU WANT DAY (see pages 100–101)

Lunch

EAT WHAT YOU WANT DAY

Dinner

EAT WHAT YOU WANT DAY
(Your favorite seafood, chicken, or lamb dish)

FIRST WEEK—SATURDAY

Breakfast

Instant Breakfast: Honeydew melon, watermelon, or grapes (as
  much as you want)

Lunch

Japanese Noodle Soup

Dinner

Popeye Salad
Green Beans with Tomatoes
Pea Pods with Basil

FIRST WEEK—SUNDAY

EAT WHAT YOU WANT (see pages 100–101)—SUNDAY
  BRUNCH
Go for it!

SECOND WEEK—MONDAY

Breakfast

Energy Plate

> Apples, peeled, cored, and sliced
> Pears, peeled, cored, and sliced
> Grapes
> Raisins, currants, or dates

  Attractively arrange apples, pears, and grapes on a plate with
dried fruit in the center.

Lunch

Romaine Wraps

Dinner

Green Goddess Salad
Millet burgers
Baked parsnips

SECOND WEEK—TUESDAY

Breakfast

Tropical Salad
_____

    Pineapple, peeled and chopped
    Grapefruit, peeled, membrane removed, and chopped
    Oranges, peeled and chopped
    3–4 oz. almonds, walnuts, pecans, filberts, or pumpkin or
       sunflower seeds

    Mix pineapple, grapefruit, and oranges in a bowl. Have nuts
or seeds on the side.

Lunch

Vegetable Sandwich

Dinner

Prize Salad
Baked sweet or white potato, or salmon, swordfish, or halibut steak
    with stuffed tomatoes
Brussels sprouts

SECOND WEEK—WEDNESDAY

Breakfast

Instant Breakfast: Oranges, watermelon, or grapefuit (as much as
    you want)

Lunch

Lentil Soup

Dinner

Venetian Salad
Cressed Carrots
Zucchini Gondolas

SECOND WEEK—THURSDAY

EAT WHAT YOU WANT DAY (see pages 100–101)

SECOND WEEK—FRIDAY

Breakfast

Grain Morning: cream of rye, millet, or oatmeal

Lunch

Caribbean Bowl

Dinner

Carrot juice
California Health Salad
Hearty Garden Stew

SECOND WEEK—SATURDAY

EAT WHAT YOU WANT DAY (see pages 100–101)

SECOND WEEK—SUNDAY

Breakfast

Fruit Plate
_____

      Pineapple, sliced
      Apple, peeled, cored, and sliced
      Grapes

      On a plate, attractively arrange as much fruit as desired.

Lunch

Oriental Express
Mediterranean Peppers
Whole-grain bread

Dinner

Sun Salad
Rice Pilaf
Mom's Beets, or grated raw beets

THIRD WEEK—MONDAY

Breakfast

Summer Plate
_____

      Blueberries
      Raspberries
      Peaches, peeled and sliced
      Grated coconut

   On a plate, attractively arrange as much fruit as desired and garnish with coconut.

Lunch

Carrot juice
Greek Salad

Dinner

Spring Salad
Corn on the cob with butter
Green Beans Dilly Delight
Corn bread

THIRD WEEK—TUESDAY

Breakfast

Grain Morning: granola with apple juice, millet, or cream of rye

Lunch

Woodstock Salad

Dinner

Easy Garden Salad
Roman Vegetables
Steamed Artichoke
Whole-grain bread

THIRD WEEK—WEDNESDAY

Breakfast

Maria's Sunny Breakfast

___

> 1 c. freshly squeezed orange juice, mixed in blender with 2
>   frozen strawberries
> Pineapple, sliced
> Apple, peeled, cored, and sliced
> 3–4 oz. almonds, pine nuts, pecans, or sunflower or sesame
>   seeds

> Attractively arrange pineapple and apple slices on a plate with
nuts or seeds in the center.

Lunch

Snappy Tomato Soup
Southern-Style Corn Bread

Dinner

John's Salad
Kasha Delight
Steamed Asparagus

THIRD WEEK—THURSDAY

Breakfast

Instant Breakfast: Watermelon, grapes, or grapefruit (as much as
    you want)

Lunch

Carrot juice
Florida Health Salad with Avocado, or
    Florida Health Salad Sandwich

Dinner
Mohican Salad
Steamed or baked potato with butter
Escarole with Oil and Garlic

THIRD WEEK—FRIDAY

EAT WHAT YOU WANT DAY (see pages 100–101)

THIRD WEEK—SATURDAY

Breakfast

Fruit Plate

        Papaya or mango, peeled and sliced
        Bing cherries
        Raspberries

        On a plate, attractively arrange as much fruit as desired.

Lunch

Rio Caliente

Dinner

Roman Salad
Zucchini Parmesan, or Broiled Lamb Chops
Steamed green beans

THIRD WEEK—SUNDAY

EAT WHAT YOU WANT DAY (see pages 100–101)

Lunch Box Menus

Monday: Plain yogurt with chopped or mashed banana,
honey, and a drop of vanilla, or plain yogurt
with fresh or frozen (sugarless) crushed
strawberries and a bit of honey
Rice crackers or cakes
Pecans or almonds
Peppermint iced tea (or any herbal tea)

Tuesday: Unsalted peanut butter and honey on whole-grain
bread
Fresh whole fruit: apple, banana, or strawberries
Green pepper and carrot sticks
Apple-grape juice or bottled coconut juice from the
health food store instead of milk

Wednesday: Sliced avocado and tomato with sprouts and a bit
of mayonnaise on whole grain bread
Semisoft cheese, cut in squares
Nuts and/or seeds and raisins or currants
Apple-grape juice or coconut juice

Thursday: Celery sticks stuffed with peanut butter
Apple
Whole wheat graham crackers

Try different bottled juices from the health food
store

Friday: Cream cheese and chopped dates on whole grain
bread
Fresh pineapple and coconut chunks
Sunflower seeds, pecans, or filberts
Apple juice

School Lunches for Kids

Everyone who raises children experiences to one degree or another
their preferences and prejudices about food. Healthful eating is
essential to a vibrant, growing body, but difficult in a TV-oriented
culture. The school cafeteria may seem an especially threatening
place, out of reach of the caring, food-conscious parent. Here in
the fogs of institutional cooking, food items are randomly traded,
and a child may be judged by the unfamiliar colors or textures hiding
in his or her lunch box. There are, however, certain guidelines that
can help lunchtime be a success, along with a little coaching and
food education at home.

Children generally favor plain foods—the basics, with no added
herbs, spices, sauces, etc.—and happily, they usually prefer raw
fruits and vegetables to cooked.

Recognizing how important it is for your child to have healthful
lunches while away from home, it is best not to be strict. Let them
have a peanut butter sandwich (fresh ground or from the health food
store) and put in a piece of fruit. It may not be the ideal combination, but it is better than having them throw out the sandwich for
a candy bar.

LUNCH BOX STAPLES

Plain yogurt
Fresh fruit in season
Coconut chunks
Nuts: almonds, walnuts,
pecans

Peanut butter—unsalted, from
the health food store
Pumpkin seeds
Sunflower seeds

DRIED FRUIT
Black currants
Raisins
Dates
Apricots

CRACKERS AND BREAD
Rye Crackers (WASA or
   similar brand)
Whole wheat graham crackers

Rice crackers or cakes
Whole grain bread

VEGETABLES
Fresh raw vegetables

DAIRY
Whipped cream cheese
Mozzarella cheese
Imported Swiss cheese

An occasional treat such as baked corn chips, puffed millet, ½ puffed millet and ½ popcorn, popcorn, or coconut-covered dates will always be appreciated. Keep a variety of fruit juices on hand. You and your child can make your own delightful combinations. Drop several slices or chunks of different fresh fruit into the juice in the Thermos occasionally for a fun surprise.

THE SUPREME (OR DISEASE-FREE) DIET

The Long Life Diet is basically a maintenance diet. It is designed to help you live healthy in a contaminated world. The Supreme Diet is based upon the Long Life Diet, but it is more healing-oriented. It is designed to help bring you back to health. It is what I call a low-stress diet, which means that your body is not forced to exert itself and use all its energy to extract the nutrients from the food you eat. On the Supreme Diet, all foods are easily digestible and easily assimilable, leaving the body with all its energy for healing purposes.

If you suffer from arthritis, hemorrhoids, constipation, general digestive problems, gastrointestinal problems, osteoporosis, heart conditions, high blood pressure, respiratory and skin conditions, eye and ear maladies, menstrual problems, menopause, or low sex drive, try the Supreme Diet. The majority of my patients with these and other problems have responded favorably over the years. My natural healing system does not treat these problems directly. But by biochemically reprogramming the body through nutrition, exercise, and dry brushing, they improve dramatically. The Supreme Diet does not pussyfoot around. You are sick and you want to get well. Stronger measures are called for.

NOTE: On the Supreme Diet, you may choose from the recipes given for the Long Life Diet and you follow the same food combining rules, but there are certain restrictions:

1. No animal protein except egg yolks is allowed. Because animal protein is kept to an absolute minimum, the body does not have to cope with uric acid buildup (see page 32).
2. "Mono day." One day of the week is devoted entirely to one of four allowable fruits. These are grapes, watermelon, apples, and grapefruit. Eat as much as you like of whatever fruit you choose. Why a mono day? A mono day is the nearest thing to fasting. Actually fasting would be better, but most people are afraid to try it or just won't do it. Fruits are the cleansers of the body and most easily digested food. When the body is not forced to work hard at digestion, it can concentrate on healing the particular problem at hand.
3. No "eat what you want" days. This may be the cruelest blow of all. The fact of the matter is, lapses from the diet when you are ill represent a step backward. This is the last thing you want. Nevertheless, I realize how difficult it is for people who are accustomed to the Standard American Diet to keep to the relative discipline of the Supreme Diet. Accordingly, I've found that when my patients put themselves on the Supreme Diet for three weeks and then relax into the Long Life Diet for one week (with its two "eat what you want" days—hurray!), little damage is done and morale improves along with health. And then it's back to the beginning of the cycle until health is restored. In other words, for the three weeks of the Supreme Diet, *no* "eat what you want" days. On the one week of the Long Life Diet, two "eat what you want" days. It's a small price to pay for good health.

NOTE: In practice, I tailor the Supreme Diet to the individual —age, lifestyle, occupation, emotional and marital status—and progress made with the individual health problem determines the specifics of the diet. Don't go overboard. Be reasonable about these fairly precise but general guidelines. Take your own situation into account and proceed accordingly.

THE WEIGHT-LOSS DIET

The Weight-Loss Diet follows the basics of the Long Life Diet, but you eat only a combination of a grapefruit and one to two stalks of celery three to four times a day, two days a week, but not on consecutive days.

I have found over the years that putting people on this combination of grapefruit and celery is a particularly powerful and healthful way to take off excess pounds. It seems that if you eat grapefruit in combination with celery, it breaks down excess fatty tissue in a way that grapefruit alone or celery alone does not. Meanwhile, the body is being purified. This same surprising combination also has a marked and beneficial sedative effect on the nervous system.

NOTE: Anything added to these grapefruit/celery days stops the process cold, even a piece of toast. You can, however, drink as much distilled water as you want. Eventually you might try three grapefruit days weekly.

CHAPTER 6

Recipes

VEGETABLES

BAKED POTATOES

Use 2–4 potatoes for 2 people, depending on size of potatoes. After scrubbing with a vegetable brush, prick with a knife and bake in a preheated 350-degree oven for 40–60 minutes, until done. If you have a toaster oven, potatoes will bake wonderfully in it. (If using a top-of-the-stove baker, cook 35–45 minutes.) Serve with sweet whipped butter.

STEAMED BROCCOLI

1 bunch broccoli
1 T. extra virgin olive oil
Juice of ¼ lemon

Trim ends off broccoli stalks. Cut broccoli into 4-in. lengths. Steam 12 minutes, until done. Drizzle with oil and lemon.

(Serves 3)

STEAMED ASPARAGUS

1 lb. asparagus
Sweet whipped butter

Wash asparagus stalks, snap off and discard the bottom ends. Tie asparagus in a neat bundle with kitchen string. Stand upright in a pot (a glass coffeepot works well) in ½ in. water and cover tightly. Bring to boil and simmer for 5 minutes, until tender. Serve with butter.

(Serves 2)

GREEN BEANS WITH TOMATOES

2 T. virgin olive oil
1 medium onion, halved lengthwise and thinly sliced
¾ c. fresh tomatoes, cubed
¾ lb. fresh green beans, cut into thirds
2 T. minced fresh oregano

Sauté oil and onion in a medium skillet over medium heat, until onion is lightly browned. Turn up heat and add tomatoes. Cook 1 minute. Add green beans and oregano, stir well, cover, and cook over low heat for 10–15 minutes, until beans are tender.

(Serves 2)

PEA PODS

¼ lb. pea pods
¼ tsp. dried basil

Wash pods. Peel back strings on each side and discard. Place pods in vegetable steamer and sprinkle with basil. Steam approximately 5 minutes, until tender.

(Serves 2)

MASHED POTATOES

Steam 2–3 medium potatoes, which have been peeled and chopped. When potatoes are tender, drain and reserve liquid. Mash potatoes with electric mixer, adding reserved liquid as needed.

BAKED PARSNIPS

1 lb. parsnips
Safflower oil

Scrub the parsnips, trim, and cut into 1¾–2-in. lengths. Coat lightly with safflower oil. Place in an iron skillet and bake in a preheated 400-degree oven until tender, about 40 minutes.

(Serves 2–3)

STUFFED TOMATOES

Remember to always serve tomato with your meat, fish, or poultry.

2 whole tomatoes, deeply cored
3 T. minced parsley
¼ c. chopped watercress
Virgin olive oil

Scoop out about ⅛ c. tomato pulp. Combine parsley and watercress, and mix with tomato pulp and enough oil to make a loose paste. Stuff the tomatoes with this mixture and cook in a preheated

400-degree oven in a covered baking dish for 20–30 minutes, until done.

(Serves 2)

BRUSSELS SPROUTS

1 lb. Brussels sprouts
Virgin olive oil
1 large onion, halved lengthwise and thinly sliced
About 3 T. water

Coat bottom of medium skillet with oil. Add onion and sauté over medium heat until slightly browned. In the meantime, wash and trim the sprouts, removing any tough outer leaves. Cut an X on the bottom. When onions are slightly browned, add Brussels sprouts, stir to mix well, add 3 T. water, and cover tightly. Simmer 20–25 minutes. Add water as needed to steam. Season with Herbamare.

(Serves 2)

ZUCCHINI GONDOLAS

2 small to medium zucchini
Cold-pressed oil
1 large onion, halved lengthwise and thinly sliced
½ lb. fresh tomatoes, peeled and diced
½ tsp. minced fresh dill
½ tsp. minced fresh oregano
½ tsp. minced fresh rosemary
1 fresh sage leaf, minced
3 T. grated Romano or Parmesan cheese
2 oz. Jarlsberg cheese, thinly sliced

Steam zucchini whole for 15 minutes, until tender. While the zucchini steam, coat a medium skillet with oil, add onion, and sauté over medium heat until onion begins to lightly brown. Turn up heat, add diced tomatoes, and cook quickly for 2 minutes. Set aside until zucchini is ready. Remove zucchini from steamer, cut in half lengthwise, and let cool. With a spoon, gently scoop out pulp, being careful not to break the outer skin. Cut the pulp into small chunks. Add zucchini pulp to onion-tomato mixture. Cook over medium heat until most of liquid evaporates. Add herbs. Turn off heat and mix in Romano or Parmesan cheese. Stuff zucchini shells with this mixture and top with Jarlsberg slices. Brown under pre-heated broiler for 5–7 minutes, until heated through and cheese begins to brown.

(Serves 2)

NOTE: This recipe can be doubled or tripled. The gondolas freeze beautifully for use in another meal. Also, you can substitute yellow squash for zucchini. For dinner parties, a mix of yellow squash and green zucchini looks very attractive.

CRESSED CARROTS

¾ lb. carrots, cut in 3-in. julienne sticks
¼ c. chopped fresh watercress or parsley
1 tsp. butter

Steam carrots about 10 minutes. Remove from steamer, and add watercress and butter.

(Serves 2)

HEARTY GARDEN STEW

1 large onion, halved lengthwise and thinly sliced
2 T. virgin olive oil
1 lb. eggplant, peeled and cut into small chunks
1 green or red bell pepper, diced
4 tomatoes, chunked, or 2½ c. canned
¾ lb. zucchini, chunked or cut into thin disks
1 celery stalk, chunked
1½ T. minced fresh oregano
1 T. fresh basil (or ½ tsp. dried)
Herbamare
Grated Parmesan or sliced Jarlsberg cheese or whole-grain
    bread

In a medium saucepan over medium heat, sauté the onion in the oil. When the onion is translucent, add the eggplant and sauté for 3 minutes. Stir often to prevent sticking. Add diced pepper and sauté for 2 minutes. Add tomatoes and bring to a boil. Cover and simmer 10 minutes over medium heat. Add zucchini, celery, oregano, and basil. Cover and simmer 10–15 minutes, until vegetables are done. Season to taste with Herbamare. This dish can be served with grated cheese or put into ovenproof dishes, topped with a few slices of Jarlsberg cheese, and put under preheated broiler until heated through and cheese is browned. If cheese is not used, serve with whole-grain bread.

(Serves 3)

MOM'S BEETS

1 bunch medium beets (4–6 beets)
Extra virgin olive oil
½ small Bermuda onion or 2 scallions, thinly sliced
3–5 fresh basil leaves, torn into pieces

Cut off beet tops, leaving 3–4 inches stem attached to beets. Scrub beets well. Steam whole 30–60 minutes, until tender (when a fork can gently be inserted). Remove from pot and allow to cool, or run under cold water. With a knife, gently peel away skins. Halve each beet and cut into thin slices. Drizzle with oil, combine with onion or scallions, and add torn fresh basil leaves. Toss. Can be served warm or cold. Remove from refrigerator 20 minutes before serving.

(Serves 2–4)

RAW GRATED BEETS

2 medium beets

Unless organically grown, peel beets. Grate on teardrop section of grater. If desired, add herbs of your choice.

(Serves 2)

CORN ON THE COB

6–8 tender ears of corn
Butter

Keep corn refrigerated until ready to cook. Husk corn and steam for 3–5 minutes, or until tender. Serve with butter.

(Serves 2–3)

GREEN BEANS DILLY DELIGHT

1 lb. tender green beans, halved
2 T. minced fresh dill
1–2 scallions, chopped
2 T. extra virgin olive oil
1 T. fresh lemon juice
½ tsp. Herbamare or Vegebase

Steam green beans until tender-crisp, about 7–10 minutes. Combine beans, dill, and scallions. In a separate bowl or jar, mix the oil, lemon juice, and Herbamare or Vegebase, until well blended. Toss into green beans. Cool slightly and serve.

(Serves 4)

ROMAN VEGETABLES

1 garlic clove, minced
¼ c. virgin olive oil
1 large ripe tomato, diced
¾ lb. green beans, cut in 4-in. pieces
1 medium zucchini, cut in quarters and chunked
1 scallion, thinly sliced, including green part
3 T. minced fresh parsley
2–3 fresh basil leaves, torn into small pieces

In a medium saucepan, sauté garlic in oil over very low heat, without browning. Turn up heat and add tomatoes. Cook for 2 minutes, uncovered. Add green beans, cover, and simmer over low heat for 10 minutes. Add zucchini, cover, and cook another 10 minutes, until vegetables are done. Remove from heat and add scallion, parsley, and basil. Cover and allow flavors to develop a few minutes before serving.

(Serves 2)

STEAMED ARTICHOKES

2 large globe artichokes
4 T. butter
3 large garlic cloves, halved lengthwise
1 T. lemon juice
Dill to taste

Select compact artichokes. Cut stem off artichoke flush with bottom. Bend back and break off the tough outer leaves. Cut 1 in. off the top of the artichoke. With kitchen shears, trim the prickly top off each leaf. Gently spread the leaves apart and pull out the choke. Wash and cook artichokes in vegetable steamer for approximately 50–60 minutes, until leaves can be easily pulled off and are tender. In the meantime, prepare sauce. In a small saucepan, melt butter over very low heat with garlic. Add lemon juice and dill. Let garlic stand in butter sauce at least 30 minutes. Heat sauce, remove garlic, and discard just before serving. Dip each leaf into sauce.

(Serves 2)

STEAMED POTATOES

2–4 medium potatoes
Sweet whipped butter

Steam potatoes for 40–60 minutes. Be sure to put enough water (about ¾ in.) in the steamer to last through the cooking process. Check water level during cooking, and add more if needed. Serve with butter.

(Serves 2)

ESCAROLE WITH OIL AND GARLIC

1 medium head of escarole
2 garlic cloves, halved lengthwise
2 T. virgin olive oil
Herbamare to taste

Wash escarole thoroughly and shake off excess water. Put escarole, garlic, and oil in a large pot. Sprinkle with Herbamare to taste. Cover tightly and let it steam with the water that remains on the escarole. Cook for 10–15 minutes, starting with moderate heat, and after it begins to steam, lower the heat. Check occasionally to be sure there is enough liquid in the pot. Remove garlic before serving.

(Serves 2)

ZUCCHINI PARMESAN

3 lbs. zucchini
2¼ lbs. tomatoes, thickly sliced
1 medium onion, thinly sliced
2 T. minced garlic
½ c. chopped fresh basil
2 T. chopped fresh oregano
1 lb. mozzarella cheese, grated
1 c. Parmesan cheese, grated

Slice zucchini diagonally ½ in. thick. Place one-third of the zucchini slices in a layer over the bottom of a large baking dish. Cover with a layer of tomato slices. Sprinkle one-third each of the onion slices, garlic, basil, and oregano over tomato layer. Cover with one-third of the grated mozzarella and about ¼ c. Parmesan. Fill the baking dish with two more layers of the remaining ingredients, reserving extra Parmesan for the top. Bake the casserole about 25 minutes in a preheated 350-degree oven, until lightly browned and bubbly.

(Serves 6)

VARIATION: In the winter this dish can be made with canned tomatoes and about ⅓ c. Basil Freeze (page 158) and 1 T. dried oregano substituted for the fresh herbs. This dish can be made ahead and reheated, and extra portions can be frozen.

STEAMED GREEN BEANS

¾ lb. green beans
Sweet whipped butter

Steam beans in vegetable steamer over moderate to low heat for 7–10 minutes, until tender. Serve with whipped butter.

(Serves 2)

VEGETABLE STIR-FRY

½ bunch broccoli
3 stalks bok choy
¼ lb. snow peas
2–3 scallions
About 2½ c. water
2 T. arrowroot
1 tsp. minced garlic
1 tsp. minced fresh ginger
2 T. tamari
1 tsp. honey
1 tsp. fresh lemon juice
1 T. black sesame oil

Begin the stir-fry by preparing all ingredients. Cut broccoli into diagonal spears; slice bok choy diagonally; trim snow peas; and slice scallions diagonally. Set all aside while preparing sauce. Pour 1½ c. water into a medium bowl. Add arrowroot and stir until dissolved. Add garlic, ginger, tamari, honey, and lemon juice. Stir and set aside. Pour enough water (about 1 c.) into wok or very large iron skillet to form a shallow pool. Add oil and place over high heat. When water begins to simmer, add broccoli. Cover for about 2 minutes and steam. Remove cover and add bok choy. Continue cooking for 1 minute, stirring constantly. Add snow peas, scallions, and bean sprouts. Stir slightly. Mix the sauce very thoroughly, and pour over the vegetables. Cover and steam about 3 minutes, or until sauce has thickened and vegetables are tender-crisp. Uncover and serve immediately, over brown rice.

(Serves 4)

MEDITERRANEAN PEPPERS

These open-face sandwiches are delicious served as an accompaniment to a salad. The peppers can be served warm or at room temperature and will keep well in the refrigerator. They taste even better when cooked on a barbecue grill.

    2 red bell peppers
    ½ T. virgin olive oil
    1 garlic clove, cut in 3 pieces
    1 T. chopped fresh parsley
    2 slices whole-grain bread

Put peppers under a preheated broiler fairly close to flame and cook until they are limp and blackened, turning often, about 20 minutes. (They are easier to peel when blackened.) Remove from broiler and place in a brown paper bag, twisting the top so they steam for a few minutes. Scrape the skin from the peppers with the blade of a sharp knife, cut in thick slices, and remove stem, seeds, and membrane. Drizzle peppers with oil and toss with garlic and parsley. Serve on slices of whole-grain bread as an open-face sandwich.

(Serves 2)

GRAINS

Breakfast cereals, such as granola or muesli, can be nutritionally improved by adding ground or chopped almonds, walnuts, or filberts. They add protein value and make a pleasant crunchy contrast to the smooth texture of the cereal. Rough chopping of nuts can be done with a knife. For finer grinding, put them through a Moulinex grinder, available in any health food or gourmet store.

OATMEAL

⅓ c. oatmeal
1 c. water
1 pat sweet whipped butter (optional)

Add oatmeal to boiling water. Cook 5 minutes, covered, stirring occasionally. Remove from heat and let stand, covered, a few minutes. Serve with butter.

(Serves 1)

CREAM OF RYE

⅓ c. cream of rye
1 c. water
1 pat sweet whipped butter (optional)

Slowly stir rye flakes into boiling water. Cook 3 minutes, covered. Turn off heat and let stand for 3 minutes. Serve with butter.

(Serves 1)

GOOD-MORNING MILLET

⅓ c. millet
1 c. apple juice or water
1 tsp. sweet whipped butter (optional)
2–8 dried currants (best to soak overnight in water)

Combine millet and liquid in a small heavy saucepan. Cover and set over medium heat. Allow to come to a simmer. Lower heat and simmer, covered, for about 20 minutes, or until all the liquid is absorbed. Add butter and currants if desired, and eat while hot.

(Serves 1)

COOKED MILLET

1½ c. millet
3 c. cold water

Combine the millet and water in a medium saucepan. Cover, place over medium heat, and bring to a boil. Quickly reduce heat and simmer about 20 minutes, until liquid is absorbed.

NOTE: Uncooked millet makes an excellent base for homemade granola and also adds body and value to soup or broth when sprinkled on after cooking or just before serving.

MILLET BURGERS

3½ c. Cooked Millet (see preceding recipe)
1 large onion, chopped
1 c. mashed potatoes (see Note)
¼ c. fresh parsley or 1 T. minced fresh dill
1½ tsp. minced garlic
3 T. whole wheat flour
Safflower oil for basting
8 whole-grain buns or 16 slices whole-grain bread (optional)
Tomato slices (optional)
Avocado slices (optional)
Tomato-Green Pepper Relish (page 159) (optional)
Tomato-Paprika Sauce (pages 159–60) (optional)

Combine the first six ingredients, mixing well. Wet hands and form the mixture into balls about 3 in. in diameter. Flatten to form patties on an oiled broiler pan or baking sheet. Brush tops with oil and place in preheated broiler. Broil about 8 minutes on each side (after turning, brush with oil), until crispy, golden brown. Serve hot millet burgers on buns or on thick slices of whole-grain bread. Top each with a slice of tomato or avocado, and Tomato-Pepper Relish or Tomato-Paprika Sauce. Unused patties can be individually wrapped and frozen. These patties are delicious served cold the next day.

(Makes 8 patties)

NOTE: Use potatoes from Vegetable Broth (page 152) or make them fresh (page 123).

RICE PILAF

> 2 T. virgin olive oil
> 8 large shallots, peeled
> 1 clove garlic, minced
> 1 large green or red bell pepper, diced
> 1 fresh plum tomato, chopped
> ½ c. fresh lemon juice (about 2 lemons)
> 2½ c. water
> 1½ c. brown rice
> ½ c. minced fresh mint
> ½ c. chopped fresh parsley

Put olive oil in a Dutch oven. Cut shallots in half. Heat oil and add shallots and pepper and sauté. Add garlic and sauté about 2 minutes (do not brown), then remove all from the pot with a slotted spoon, reserving as much of the juices as possible. Set vegetables aside. Put tomato, lemon juice, water, and rice into the pot. Cover and bring to a simmer. Cook, covered, for 45 minutes, or until the rice absorbs all the liquid. When the rice is cooked, stir in herbs and sautéed shallot-pepper mixture, and serve. Leftover Rice Pilaf can be refrigerated and served another time cold on a bed of crisp lettuce. Rice pilaf can also be frozen and thawed in the oven for a quick supper.

BROWN RICE

> 1 c. long-grain brown rice
> 2 c. water

Put water and rice in a pot with a tight-fitting cover. Bring to a boil, cover, and simmer 40 minutes. (Don't peek.) After 40 min-

utes, turn off heat and let the rice set a few minutes. Fluff with a
fork.

Serves 3–4)

KASHA DELIGHT

4 T. virgin olive oil
1½ c. buckwheat groats
3 c. boiling water mixed with 1 T. Vegebase
2 large onions, coarsely chopped
2 tsp. paprika
2 T. fresh thyme or 1 tsp. dried
1½ c. fresh peas or chopped spinach
Herbamare to taste

Heat 1 T. of oil in a medium iron skillet or Dutch oven. Pour
in the groats and toss in the oil until lightly toasted, about 4 minutes.
Reduce heat and slowly pour in the boiling water and Vegebase.
Cover and simmer until groats are cooked, about 20 minutes. Meanwhile, heat remaining 3 T. of oil in a large skillet. Add the chopped
onions and sauté slowly, until transparent. Add paprika and thyme.
Add cooked kasha and blend well with the onions and seasonings.
Add peas or spinach and toss. Turn off heat. Cover pot for about
2 minutes, allowing vegetables to steam in the hot kasha until peas
are tender-crisp or spinach slightly wilted. Remove cover immediately and season with Herbamare or additional Vegebase to taste.
Freeze any unused kasha.

(Serves 4–6)

NUTS

There are endless variations of nut cutlets, nut burgers, nut
patties, soups, sauces, etc., all using chopped nuts in combination
with vegetables, flour, rice, herbs, onion, and seasonings. Ask your
health food store owner about nut recipe books.

FRUIT AND VEGETABLE SALADS, SOUPS, SANDWICHES, AND CORNBREAD

AVOCADO VEGETABLE BOWL

If you're really hungry you can add any other fresh vegetables you'd like, such as fresh peas or bok choy.

1 avocado, chunked
1 tomato, chunked
½ red or green bell pepper, sliced
1 small cucumber, peeled and chunked
½ c. alfalfa sprouts or a few sprigs watercress
2–3 fresh basil leaves, minced
1 T. sunflower, corn, black sesame, or extra virgin
    olive oil
Lemon juice to taste

Mix all the ingredients in a bowl except oil and lemon juice. Then toss with oil and lemon juice.

(Serves 1)

FRUIT DELIGHT

½–1 avocado, sliced
3–4 leaves romaine lettuce
1–2 bananas, cut in thick slices
2–3 peaches, sliced
1 apple or Bosc pear, chunked
Apple juice to taste

Arrange avocado slices on lettuce around the rim of a plate. In between the avocado slices add banana and peach slices. Put apple or pear chunks in the center of plate and drizzle apple juice over the fruit.

(Serves 1)

NOTE: This mixture of lettuce with fruit is permissible.

CARROT WALDORF SALAD

1 large carrot
3 T. Homemade Mayonnaise (page 162)
2 tsp. lemon juice
1 celery or bok choy stalk, sliced
1 large apple, peeled, cored, and diced
¼ c. pecan or walnut pieces
1 head Bibb lettuce

Grind the carrot as fine as possible in food processor or blender. Mix with mayonnaise and lemon juice. In another bowl combine the celery, apple, and pecans or walnuts. Toss everything with the carrot-mayonnaise mixture. Serve the salad heaped in the center of a bed of Bibb lettuce leaves.

(Serves 2)

NOTE: The apple in this mixture of vegetables is permissible.

ROMAINE WRAP

3–4 large leaves romaine lettuce
6–8 cherry tomatoes, halved
2 celery stalks, sliced
1 carrot, grated
1 cucumber, peeled and chopped
3 oz. imported Swiss, French feta, ricotta, or cottage cheese
Salad dressing

Lay out lettuce leaves and divide up remaining vegetables and cheese onto the center of each leaf. Top with salad dressing. Wrap each leaf around the filling.

(Serves 1)

CARIBBEAN BOWL

½–1 avocado, cut in chunks
½ pint strawberries, halved
1 grapefruit, sectioned, and juiced (optional),
    or ½ papaya (optional)
Apple juice (optional)
Shredded coconut
Fresh mint (optional)

Mix together avocado, strawberries, and grapefruit or papaya. Drizzle with apple juice *only* if papaya is substituted for grapefruit. Garnish with coconut and mint.

(Serves 1)

GREEK SALAD

½ head of Bibb, Boston, or romaine lettuce
2 carrots, sliced
2 celery stalks, sliced
1 cucumber, peeled and sliced
1 stalk bok choy, sliced
½ c. bean sprouts
3 oz. French feta cheese
Salad dressing

Mix the first six ingredients together. Break the feta cheese into chunks and add to salad. Add your favorite salad dressing and toss.

(Serves 1)

SUNNY SPINACH SALAD

¾–1 lb. spinach leaves, packed, cleaned, trimmed, and torn
3 large leaves romaine lettuce, torn into large pieces
2 stalks celery, chopped
1 white or red radish, sliced
1 Sunny Carrot Dip (page 163)

Combine the spinach and romaine leaves in a large bowl with chopped celery and radish slices. Toss. Arrange the salad mixture on individual plates. Mound the Sunny Carrot Dip in the center of each serving.

(Serves 2)

RED-LEAF AVOCADO SALAD

The avocado dressing makes an excellent dip for raw vegetables.

½ avocado
½ c. chopped fresh parsley
2 T. lemon juice
3 T. extra virgin olive oil
1 tsp. raw honey
1 large head red-leaf lettuce
1 medium beet, peeled and grated
1 scallion, thinly sliced

Combine avocado, parsley, lemon juice, olive oil, and honey in blender or food processor. Blend until smooth. Set aside. Wash and trim lettuce. Break into bite-size pieces. Arrange on individual salad plates, garnished with grated beet and sliced scallion. Spoon avocado dressing into center of plate.

(Serves 3)

GREEN GODDESS SALAD

8 oz. Boston lettuce
2 oz. spinach
½ c. watercress
2 celery stalks, sliced
2 Jerusalem artichokes, sliced
½ avocado, chunked
2 carrots, grated
Salad dressing

Tear Boston lettuce, spinach, and watercress into bite-size pieces. Mix with celery, Jerusalem artichokes, and avocado. Top with grated carrots and salad dressing.

(Serves 2)

POPEYE SALAD

6 oz. spinach
2 oz. leaf lettuce
½ c. watercress
2 oz. Chinese cabbage, thinly sliced
1 cucumber, peeled and sliced
½ red bell pepper
½ green bell pepper
½ avocado, sliced
Salad dressing

Tear the spinach, lettuce, and watercress into bite-size pieces. Mix with remaining vegetables and toss with your favorite dressing.

(Serves 2)

DR. JACK'S GARDEN SALAD

8 oz. red-leaf lettuce
2 small beets, peeled and grated
2 stalks bok choy, sliced
2 Jerusalem artichokes, sliced
2 thin slices Bermuda onion (optional)
1 sheet nori seaweed, broken into pieces
2 carrots, sliced
1 tsp. uncooked millet
Salad dressing

Tear lettuce into bite-size pieces. Mix with next six ingredients and toss. Divide between serving plates, sprinkle ½ teaspoon millet onto each serving, and add dressing.

(Serves 2)

PRIZE SALAD

12 oz. romaine lettuce
2 cucumbers, peeled and sliced
2 carrots, sliced
1 red bell pepper, sliced
1 c. alfalfa sprouts
Salad dressing

Tear lettuce into bite-size pieces. Mix with next four ingredients. Toss with dressing.

(Serves 2)

PLAZA SALAD

10 oz. Bibb lettuce
2 oz. red cabbage, shredded
2 carrots, sliced
1 cucumber, peeled and sliced
½ avocado, sliced
1 scallion, thinly sliced
Salad dressing

Tear lettuce into bite-size pieces, combine with remaining ingredients, and toss.

(Serves 2)

CALIFORNIA HEALTH SALAD

8 oz. red-leaf lettuce
2 oz. romaine lettuce
2 oz. Chinese cabbage, thinly shredded
1 cucumber, peeled and sliced
2 Jerusalem artichokes, sliced
2 carrots, grated
½ c. mung bean sprouts
Salad dressing

Tear lettuces into bite-size pieces. Mix with next four ingredients, and toss with dressing. Divide between serving plates and top each portion with ¼ c. sprouts.

(Serves 2)

VENETIAN SALAD

4 oz. spinach
4 oz. Bibb lettuce
4 oz. red cabbage, thinly sliced
¼ c. chopped watercress
2 tomatoes, cut in large chunks
1 cucumber, peeled and sliced
1 Jerusalem artichoke, thinly sliced
Salad dressing

Tear spinach and lettuce into bite-size pieces. Combine with cabbage, watercress, tomatoes, cucumber, and Jerusalem artichoke. Toss with dressing and serve.

(Serves 2)

SUN SALAD

8 oz. romaine lettuce
4 oz. spinach
2 oz. red cabbage, thinly sliced
1 cucumber, peeled and chunked
1 carrot, sliced
½ avocado, sliced
1 c. mung bean sprouts
Salad dressing

Tear lettuce and spinach into bite-size pieces. Mix with cabbage, cucumber, carrot, and avocado. Toss with dressing. Divide between serving plates and top each portion with ½ c. bean sprouts.

(Serves 2)

SPRING SALAD

10 oz. red-leaf lettuce
2 oz. red cabbage, thinly sliced
¼ c. cooked chick peas
1 red bell pepper, sliced
2 carrots, sliced
2 celery stalks, chopped
Salad dressing

Tear lettuce into bite-size pieces. Mix with next five ingredients and toss with dressing.

(Serves 2)

EASY GARDEN SALAD

8 oz. romaine lettuce
2 stalks bok choy, thinly sliced
2 thin slices Bermuda onion
2 celery stalks, chopped
½ avocado, chopped
Salad dressing
1 c. alfalfa sprouts

Tear lettuce into bite-size pieces. Mix with next four ingredients. Toss with dressing. Divide between serving plates, placing ½ c. sprouts on the center of each portion.

(Serves 2)

JOHN'S SALAD

6 oz. Boston lettuce
4 oz. leaf lettuce
2 carrots, sliced
2 celery stalks, sliced
2 Jerusalem artichokes, sliced
2 cucumbers, peeled and sliced
1 c. mung bean sprouts
Salad dressing

Tear lettuce into bite-size pieces and combine with next five ingredients. Toss with salad dressing.

(Serves 2)

MOHICAN SALAD

6 oz. Boston lettuce
4 oz. spinach
2 oz. red cabbage, shredded
2 carrots, grated
1 cucumber, peeled and sliced
½ avocado, sliced
Salad dressing

Tear lettuce and spinach into bite-size pieces. Add cabbage, carrots, cucumber, and avocado. Toss with dressing.

(Serves 2)

ROMAN SALAD

6 oz. romaine lettuce
2 oz. arugula
2 carrots, sliced
2 tomatoes, chopped
1 celery stalk, sliced
Salad dressing
2 c. alfalfa sprouts

Tear lettuce and arugula into bite-size pieces. Add next three ingredients. Toss with dressing. Divide between serving plates and top each serving with 1 c. sprouts.

(Serves 2)

WOODSTOCK SALAD

1 grapefruit, peeled, sectioned, and chunks removed (be sure to squeeze out all the sweet juice)
½–1 avocado, cut in chunks
1–2 apples, peeled, cored, and chopped
Fresh mint (optional)

Mix together first three ingredients. Garnish with mint.

(Serves 1)

RIO CALIENTE

6 leaves romaine lettuce
1 cucumber, cut in julienne sticks
1 celery stalk, cut in julienne sticks
1 carrot, cut in julienne sticks
8 cherry tomatoes
½ avocado
1 small tomato, peeled

Arrange lettuce leaves on a platter and top with the next four ingredients. In a blender, mix avocado with small peeled tomato. Pour into center of platter. Dip vegetables and lettuce into tomato and avocado mixture or toss as a salad.

(Serves 1)

FLORIDA HEALTH SALAD WITH AVOCADO
(OR FLORIDA HEALTH SALAD SANDWICH)

This will also make a tasty spread for crackers or sandwiches.

2 c. grated carrots (see NOTE)
¼ c. mayonnaise
1 celery stalk, diced
¼ c. chopped watercress or 3 T. minced fresh parsley
1 T. minced scallion or onion
¼ tsp. minced fresh dill
1 avocado, halved, or 4 slices whole-grain bread
4 large leaves lettuce
1 cucumber, sliced

Mix together the first six ingredients and divide between the centers of the avocado halves, on a bed of lettuce, or serve as a sandwich on whole-grain bread with lettuce leaves. Serve with cucumber slices.

(Serves 2)

NOTE: If you have a juicer you can substitute 1 c. pulp from juiced carrots for the 2 c. grated carrots, and add 2 Tb. more mayonnaise to recipe.

ORIENTAL EXPRESS

½ head leaf lettuce
1 celery stalk
1 radish, thinly sliced
1 stalk bok choy
¼ c. mung bean sprouts
2 thin slices Bermuda onion
Salad dressing

Mix all the vegetables together and add salad dressing.

(Serves 1)

SNAPPY TOMATO SOUP

Sesame oil
1 large onion, cut in half lengthwise and thinly sliced
1 green bell pepper, diced
2 lbs. tomatoes, diced
1 celery stalk, chopped
15–20 green beans, cut in thirds
2 sq. in. Basil Freeze (page 158) (optional)
1½ tsp. Vegebase
Fresh or dried herbs to taste, such as basil, parsley, and
    oregano
2 large tomatoes, peeled and quartered
Herbamare to taste

Coat bottom of stock-pot with oil, and sauté onion over low heat. When browned, sauté green pepper for 2 minutes. Add 2 lbs. tomatoes and cover. Cook 10 minutes over medium to high heat. Add celery and green beans, cover, and cook until vegetables are done, about 10 minutes. Add Basil Freeze, Vegebase, and herbs. Put quartered raw tomatoes into blender with 2½ c. soup and purée. Mix with the remaining soup and reheat just before serving. Season to taste with Herbamare.

(Serves 2)

LENTIL SOUP

1 medium onion, halved lengthwise and thinly sliced
⅛ c. sesame oil
1 c. dried lentils, washed
1 qt. boiling water
1 celery stalk, chopped
2 carrots, chopped
1 tomato, chopped
1 T. Vegebase
2 sq. in. Basil Freeze (page 158) (optional)
Fresh dill to taste
¼ c. chopped watercress
1 tsp. butter
Herbamare to taste

In a stockpot, sauté onion in oil until translucent. Add washed lentils and sauté for 2 minutes. Add water, cover, and simmer 45 minutes, until lentils are tender. Add celery, carrots, tomato, Vegebase, Basil Freeze, and dill, and cook 10 minutes. Put 3 c. of soup in blender and purée. Return to pot, add watercress and butter, and heat through. Season to taste with Herbamare.

(Serves 2–4)

SUSAN'S CREAMY POTATO-CABBAGE SOUP

This very special recipe came to me via Susan Jezierski, who is a wonderful vegetarian gourmet cook. This truly tasty meal will help you overcome your meat-and-potatoes habit.

1 medium onion, thinly sliced
¼ c. sesame oil
¼ tsp. caraway seed
¼ medium head green cabbage, cut in half and thinly sliced
2 carrots, sliced
4 medium potatoes, peeled and quartered
4 c. water
1 tsp. butter
2 tsp. Vegebase
Watercress or parsley, chopped
Herbamare to taste

In a stockpot, sauté onion in sesame oil over medium heat. When onion is translucent, add caraway seed and cabbage and sauté 2 minutes. Add carrots, potatoes, and water. Bring to a boil, cover, and simmer 20–25 minutes. Remove 4 c. of vegetables, put them in a blender, and purée. Return purée to pot. Just before serving, add butter, Vegebase, and a handful of chopped watercress or parsley. Season to taste with Herbamare.

(Serves 2)

NOTE: Sometimes cooked cabbage tends to create gas. The caraway seed neutralizes that effect.

JAPANESE NOODLE SOUP

3 c. Vegetable Broth (see following recipe)
1 carrot, diced
1 celery stalk, diced
1 scallion, sliced
½ tsp. fresh dill or parsley or ¼ c. chopped watercress
2½ oz. Japanese bean or soy noodles, or other thin pasta
Herbamare to taste

Bring the Vegetable Broth to a boil. Add the carrot and celery. Cover, bring to a boil, and simmer about 10 minutes, until vegetables are almost done. Turn up heat and add the scallion, dill or parsley or watercress, and noodles. Stir to break the noodles apart. Simmer, covered, until noodles are done, about 3 minutes. Serve immediately. This soup should not sit long after being cooked because noodles will absorb the broth.

(Serves 2)

VEGETABLE BROTH

4 large potatoes, peeled and cut into eighths
2 large carrots, cut into 1-in. pieces
2 celery stalks, cut into 1-in. pieces
1 small zucchini, cut into 1-in. pieces (optional)
About 5 c. water

In a 4-qt. stockpot, place the first four ingredients. Cover with water (this will be approximately 5 c.). Cover pot and bring to boil over medium heat. Simmer until potatoes are fork tender, approximately 35 minutes. Strain broth, reserving whatever vegetables you'd enjoy eating. This broth will keep in the refrigerator for several days, or it can be made in large batches and frozen.

(Serves 2 as a main dish or use as a snack)

NOTE: You can make mashed potatoes from the potatoes in this broth. Reserve potatoes, add 2 pats of butter and ¼ c. of broth, and mix with electric beater until fluffy and smooth. Add more broth if needed. You'll have light, fluffy, and delicious mashed potatoes. To reheat the mashed potatoes, simply add heated broth to them and mash again with a fork. You can also use these mashed potatoes in the millet burger recipe (page 134).

VEGETABLE SANDWICH

Whipped butter or cold-pressed mayonnaise
2 slices sourdough rye, soy, or whole-grain bread
½ cucumber, sliced lengthwise
2 thick slices of tomato
1 lettuce leaf
Watercress to taste
1 carrot, cut lengthwise in sticks, for garnish

Spread butter or mayonnaise on one side of each slice of bread. Layer the sliced vegetables on one slice of bread in the order listed and top with the other slice of bread. Have carrot sticks on the side.

(Serves 1)

THE GREAT MOHICAN

This sandwich is named after one of the oldest fruit and vegetable markets in the country, the Mohican Fruit and Vegetable Market in Kingston, New York. You should search out a specialty market in your area that features fresh organic produce. This is a great sandwich to take to work, on a picnic, or on a trip to the beach.

Homemade Mayonnaise (page 162)
2 slices sourdough rye, soy, or whole-grain bread
¼ avocado, sliced
2 thick slices of tomato
1 oz. alfalfa sprouts
Watercress
1 leaf romaine lettuce
1 carrot or celery stalk, for garnish

Spread mayonnaise on one side of each slice of bread. Place sliced avocado, tomato slices, sprouts, watercress, and romaine lettuce on one slice of bread and top with the other slice. Serve with cucumber or carrot sticks on the side.

(Serves 1)

CORN BREAD

This delicious corn bread is another recipe from *The Vegan Kitchen* cookbook (see page 103).

Mix:
¼ c. soy powder
½ c. water
1 tsp. tahini
1 T. oil
1 mashed banana

Mix:
1½ c. cornmeal
1 c. water

Stir two mixtures together. Pour into oiled loaf pan or oiled muffin pans. Bake in a preheated 400-degree oven for 45 minutes.

SOUTHERN-STYLE CORN BREAD

Excellent corn bread mixes are often available from Arrowhead Mills through your health food store. If you don't see them, ask for them. Walnut Acres has an excellent mix and a mail-order catalog. (See mail-order list at the back of book for address.)

POULTRY, FISH, LAMB, AND PASTA

CHICKEN OREGANATO

3 T. chopped fresh parsley
2 T. fresh oregano or 2 tsp. dried
⅓ c. virgin olive oil
The juice of 1 lemon
1 garlic clove, minced
One 2½-lb. chicken, quartered
2 tomatoes, cut in thick slices

Mix parsley, oregano, oil, lemon juice, and garlic together. Marinate chicken in this mixture for 20 minutes or longer. Place chicken pieces in a preheated broiler about 6 in. from the flame. Broil 15–20 minutes on each side, turning once, until brown and tender. Baste occasionally with marinade. Serve with tomato slices.

(Serves 2)

BROILED FISH

2 salmon, swordfish, or halibut steaks
2 lemons
Virgin olive oil
Fresh dill

Wash steaks well in cold water and pat dry with paper towels. Rub surfaces with ½ lemon, wash steaks again, and dry on paper towels. Prepare a marinade with oil, dill, and 2 T. lemon juice. Put fish steaks into marinade for 20 minutes, turning them a few times. Cook in a preheated broiler for 5–6 minutes on each side, until they can be flaked with a fork. Serve with remaining lemon cut into wedges.

(Serves 2)

BROILED LAMB CHOPS

2–4 lamb chops
1 tsp. dried rosemary
1 garlic clove, cut into 4 pieces
2–3 T. virgin olive oil
4 lemon wedges
1 tomato, cut in thick slices

Being careful not to make a deep incision in the meat, insert a chunk of garlic in each chop next to the bone. Marinate in oil and rosemary for about 10 minutes. Cook in a preheated broiler, turning once for 5 minutes on each side, until done. Serve with lemon wedges and tomato slices.

(Serves 2)

PASTA À LA RICHARD

Here is one of the simplest and best of pastas, from noted goldsmith and gourmet cook, Richard Messina. It can be prepared in the time it takes you to kick off your shoes, boil water, and cook the pasta.

2 T. extra virgin olive oil
2 garlic cloves, peeled and halved
¾ lb. zucchini, grated (about 3 c.)
2 Tb. sweet whipped butter
¼ tsp. Herbamare or Vegebase
½ lb. Jerusalem artichoke pasta

Put olive oil in a medium skillet and slowly heat with garlic. When garlic becomes soft, gently crush it with the back of a fork, and cook until lightly golden—do not brown. Turn up heat, add zucchini, and cook until liquid begins to come out, about 3 minutes. Add Herbamare or Vegebase. Remove garlic before serving. Cook pasta according to package directions, drain, and place in a bowl. Cover with zucchini mixture.

(Serves 2)

NOTE: This recipe without the pasta makes an excellent zucchini side dish for any meal.

HERBS, SPICES, AND SEASONINGS

FOR SALADS AND VEGETABLES	FOR FISH	FOR POULTRY
basil	dill	marjoram
caraway seed	fennel	mint
dill	garlic	onion
garlic	marjoram	oregano
onion	mint	parsley
oregano	onion	rosemary
parsley	parsley	sage
rosemary	rosemary	tarragon
sage	sage	thyme
tarragon	thyme	Herbamare
thyme	Herbamare	

Herbamare (sea salt and dried herbs)
   from health food store
Vegebase (Vogue) from health food store

Since freshness and quality are now being recognized as important, more and more supermarkets and vegetable markets are carrying fresh herbs such as dill, parsley, oregano, thyme, rosemary, and basil throughout the year. These herbs can be washed and frozen and ready for use at a moment's notice. Just remove from freezer and chop off the amount you need and return to the freezer for next time. They make wonderful additions to your meals without being any extra bother.

   If you are substituting dried herbs for fresh ones, remember that dried herbs are concentrated and therefore more potent, and so should be ¼ to ½ of what the recipe calls for with fresh herbs.

   When garlic is called for in a recipe, put the clove on a hard surface. Lay the flat side of a heavy knive blade on it and strike firmly with your other hand to smash the garlic. This will release the flavor and make peeling the skin easier.

BASIL FREEZE

With the increasing popularity of basil, which appears in many dishes from pasta to potatoes, here is an excellent way to store the garden-fresh herb at its peak in mid- to late summer for culinary pleasure through the winter months.

    3 c. chopped fresh basil leaves
    ½ c. extra virgin olive oil

Process basil in processor or blender (half at a time, if necessary) with oil until puréed. Measure about ½ c. into half-pint Ziploc freezer storage bags. Press the purée flat, filling the bag to within ⅛ in. of the closing. Close the bags and freeze them on flat trays or on the bottom shelf of the freezer. When they are frozen, the bags can be conveniently stacked. For use in soups, sauces, salad dressings, etc., just break off small pieces of the frozen sheet (2 sq. in. equals about 1 T. minced basil), reseal bag, and return to freezer.

    (Makes 2 c.)

PESTO

    ½–1 garlic clove
    1½ T. pine nuts
    ½ pt. Basil Freeze (see preceding recipe)
    ¼ c. grated Parmesan cheese

Put garlic and pine nuts with Basil Freeze in blender. Mix thoroughly and remove. Add Parmesan cheese. Serve as a sauce for pasta on your "eat what you want" day.

VARIATION: Mix 1½ c. pesto with ½ c. sour cream to make a dressing for a baked potato, crisp steamed broccoli, or fresh raw tomatoes.

TOMATO-GREEN PEPPER RELISH

½ red onion, quartered
1 large green bell pepper, quartered
½ c. chopped parsley
2 tsp. minced garlic
2 tsp. lemon juice
1 large tomato, quartered

Using a large wooden chopping bowl or broad salad bowl and a crescent-shaped blade, chop the onion quite small. Add the pepper pieces, parsley, and garlic, and continue chopping until the pepper is well minced. Add the lemon juice and tomato, and continue to chop until the tomato is minced and all ingredients are well mixed.

(Makes 2 c.)

NOTE: A food processor may be used to make this relish, pulsing one at a time the onion, green pepper, tomato, and parsley, to make a uniformly fine texture, without totally pulverizing. The use of the chopping bowl and blade is suggested here as a good way to preserve the individuality of the ingredients yet allow a thorough mixing of flavors.

AVOCADO JUBILEE

Stuff Tomato-Green Pepper Relish (see preceding recipe) into avocado halves for a spectacular first course.

TOMATO-PAPRIKA SAUCE

1 medium onion, chopped
2 T. virgin olive oil
1 T. chopped garlic
5 plum tomatoes, peeled and chopped (see NOTE)
2 T. chopped fresh parsley
2 tsp. paprika
3 tsp. fresh lemon juice

In a small saucepan over medium-low heat, gently sauté onions in oil until golden. Add garlic and brown very slightly, continually stirring. Add tomatoes and simmer 4 minutes. Add parsley and paprika. Simmer about 2 more minutes, then stir in lemon juice. Serve sauce hot with bean dishes or hot or cold with grain patties.

(Makes 1½ c.)

NOTE: Dip tomatoes into boiling water for 30 seconds, then slip off the skins. Canned tomatoes may be substituted.

DRINKS, DRESSINGS, SNACKS, AND DIPS

FRESHLY MADE JUICES

Purchasing a juicer is wise, not only for the tasty juices you can make with it but for the even greater benefit that the juices have on your overall health. It's fun to serve these as cocktails while you're preparing your meal. It's best to let 20–30 minutes lapse from the time you have your juice until you eat anything. Be sure to drink the juice slowly, savoring every mouthful.

FRUIT SHAKES

To turn any shake into a cholesterol killer, add 1 rounded tsp. lecithin granules. This helps dissolve cholesterol.

⅓ c. yogurt
1–2 bananas or 2–3 peaches or 1 banana and 1–2 peaches
   (peel all fruit)
⅛ c. apple juice (optional, for thinner shakes)

Mix all ingredients in blender until well blended. The consistency can be thin enough to drink or thick enough to eat with a spoon.

(Serves 1)

VARIATION: Try adding 1 tsp. sesame tahini or grated coconut or both to any shake.

VARIATION: Make up your own shakes with any fruit in season. For example:
    nectarines (peeled) and blueberries
    or
    peaches (peeled) and grapes
    or
    fresh pineapple chunks and grapes or berries

Use as much fruit as you'd like, plus:
⅛ cup apple juice
1 rounded tsp. lecithin granules or 1 tsp.
    sesame tahini

Mix in blender to desired consistency.

HIGH-PROTEIN POWER DRINK

2 heaping T. unsalted soy nuts
1 T. currants
3 T. fresh grated coconut
1 tsp. lecithin granules
4–6 oz. apple juice (to taste)

Blend all ingredients together.

MARIA'S DELIGHT

Maria Del Tondo from Danbury, Connecticut uses this easy-to-make and delicious drink to quench the thirst of family and friends during hot summer months.

Brew herbal lemon iced tea and herbal orange iced tea according to package directions. Combine, using equal parts of each.

Chill. Serve with fresh mint, thin lemon slices, and thin orange slices. Honey may be added to taste.

MARIA'S SUN TEA

During the summer, Maria Del Tondo makes sun tea: Put 3–4 herbal tea bags in a 1-qt. Mason jar (or any clear glass bottle). Fill with 1 qt. of distilled water and cover loosely. Place jar outside in the sun or in a sunny window for 2–4 hours. Remove tea bags and chill. Serve with fresh mint.

HEALTHY SNACKS

Fresh fruit, such as: a dish of blueberries
                          watermelon
                          nectarines
                          pineapple or whatever juicy fruit you like best.
Celery sticks and nut butter *or*
Celery sticks and cottage cheese
Fresh nuts *or* seeds and dried fruits

HOMEMADE MAYONNAISE

2 egg yolks
1 T. lemon juice
1 T. hot water
¾ c. cold-pressed oil

Put the egg yolks, lemon juice, hot water, and ¼ c. oil in a blender and blend on low speed until mixed. Slowly and in a steady stream, with the blender on, add as much of remaining oil as necessary to reach desired consistency.

(Makes 1 c.)

DR. JACK'S TAHINI MAYONNAISE

¾ cup commerical cold-pressed mayonnaise (from health
  food store)
¼ cup tahini (bottled or loose, from health food store)
Juice of ¼ lemon
1–2 egg yolks (optional)

Mix all ingredients well in a blender. Store in refrigerator. Use
as a spread for sandwiches or as a salad dressing.

(Makes 1–1¼ c.)

NOTE: The tahini and lemon have a neutralizing effect on the vinegar
in commercial mayonnaise. You also get the benefit of calcium from
tahini.

SUNNY CARROT DIP

*This dip may be served with any of your favorite raw vegetables or
used as a dressing for salad greens.*

2 large carrots, chopped
6 T. extra virgin olive oil
Juice of 1 large lemon
½ small garlic clove

Place chopped carrots in food processor or blender. Grind until
texture is fairly fine and uniform. Add other ingredients and blend
until smooth. Keep unused portion refrigerated.

(Makes ¾–1 c.)

NUT BUTTERS

A nut butter spread for your toast makes a healthful change
from butter and jam. Put 2 c. nuts in your blender and grind for 1
minute to chop finely. Remove. Place ¼ c. back in your blender,

add 1 tsp. oil, and blend until creamy. Remove blender top and add balance of the ground nuts. Blend until a crunchy texture is achieved, longer for a smoother consistency. Add a little more oil if necessary. This is a gray area, not quite 100% good for you, but it's not bad when used occasionally and sparingly.

DESSERTS

COCONUT-APPLE CRISP

> 1 c. rolled oats
> ¾ c. fresh coconut, grated
> ¼ c. whole wheat flour
> ¾ c. chopped pecans or walnuts
> 1 tsp. cinnamon
> ¼ tsp. freshly grated nutmeg
> 5 T. melted butter
> ½ c. honey
> 3 very large baking apples (Rome or Ida Red)
> Safflower oil

Combine the oats, coconut, flour, nuts, and spices in a mixing bowl. Blend well. Mix the butter and honey, and pour into dry ingredients. Stir to mix thoroughly.

Thinly slice the apples. Lay slices into a lightly oiled medium baking dish (about 7 by 9 in.). Sprinkle the nut mixture evenly over the top. Bake in a preheated 400-degree oven for about 25 minutes, until browned and crusty.

(Serves 6–8)

PEACH COBBLER

Safflower oil
5 c. peeled and sliced fresh peaches (2–3 lbs.)
½ c. light honey
2 c. whole wheat pastry flour
3 tsp. non-aluminum baking powder from the health food
    store
5 T. butter
⅔–¾ cup bottled pineapple-coconut juice or apple juice

Lightly oil an 8 × 10-in. baking pan. Place prepared peaches in the pan. Add the honey and gently stir through.

Combine and sift the flour and baking powder. Cut in the butter until a mealy texture is formed. Add the juice, folding gently until all the mixture is moist but firm. Pat the dough to about ¼ in. thickness and place over the peaches in the baking pan. This can be done in sections. Set the pan in a preheated 375-degree oven and bake about 20 minutes, until golden brown on top. Serve warm.

(Serves 6)

CARROT CAKE

This delicious recipe comes from a nearby health food store, Mother Earth Storehouse, Kingston, New York.

4 eggs
1 c. clover honey
1⅓ c. melted butter
1 T. "real" vanilla
2 c. organic whole wheat flour
½ tsp. sea salt
2 T. single-acting baking powder (Rumford)
2 T. baking soda
½ tsp. nutmeg
½ tsp. cinnamon
½ tsp. cloves
½ tsp. ginger
4 cups grated carrots (about 1 lb.)
½ cup raisins
½ cup chopped walnuts

Combine eggs, honey, butter, and vanilla. Mix in flour, sea salt, baking powder, baking soda, and spices. Mix thoroughly. Fold in carrots, raisins, and walnuts. Pour into a buttered 9 × 9-in. pan. Bake 30 minutes in a preheated 350-degree oven.

(Serves 6–8)

PINEAPPLE CARROT CAKE

¾ c. finely chopped fresh pineapple with juice
¾ c. grated fresh coconut
3 c. grated carrots (about ¾ lb.)
¼ c. butter
1 c. honey
3 eggs, beaten
2 c. whole wheat pastry flour
2 tsp. baking soda
1 tsp. cinnamon
Safflower oil
8 oz. whipped cream cheese
About 3 Tb. honey

Mix chopped pineapple and its juice with the grated coconut and carrots.

Melt butter in a small saucepan. Stir in honey and eggs. Add to carrot mixture. Sift flour with soda and cinnamon. Stir into wet ingredients until well mixed. Pour batter into an oiled 9-in. tube pan. Bake in a preheated 350-degree oven for 1 hour and 10 minutes, or until an inserted tester comes out clean. Cool on a rack, then spread with cream cheese icing, if desired.

To prepare icing, whip cream cheese until light and fluffy. Slowly drizzle in honey to taste while continuing to whip.

(Serves 6–8)

FOOD DESIRABILITY INDEX

"Yes" Foods

Whole-Grain Breads, Flours, and Pasta

All sprouted grains
Millet
Rye (sourdough)
Soy
Brown rice cakes
Corn
Buckwheat
Pastas made of corn, spinach, brown rice, soy, buckwheat, or
    Jerusalem artichokes from health food store
Wasa crackers (Lite Rye)

Dried Legumes

Lentils
Chick-peas (garbanzos)
Kidney beans
Pinto beans
Lima beans (highly alkaline)
Soybeans (high protein)
Mung beans
Adzuki beans

Sweeteners

Tupelo honey
Honey (preferably dark, raw, unfiltered)
Barbados molasses
Pure maple syrup
Date sugar
Carob
NOTE: Diabetics and hypoglycemics must use caution with all
    sweeteners.

Animal Protein

Deep-sea fish
    Flounder
    Sole
    Halibut
    Red snapper
    Mackerel
    Codfish
    Swordfish
    Tuna (not canned)
    Salmon (not smoked)
    Scrod
Lamb
Fowl ("free range" only or frozen from health food store)
Eggs (yolk only, fertilized)
Calves' liver (only occasionally; no other beef)

Grains

Millet (the only alkaline cereal)
Puffed millet
Millet flakes
Buckwheat groats, or kasha
Brown rice
Cornmeal
Cream of rye
Granola
Oatmeal (Scottish, Irish, or Elam's) (on occasion)
Couscous (on occasion)
Barley (on occasion)

Dairy Products
(small portions occasionally)

Yogurt (Columbo, Lacto, Continental, Brown Cow), plain only
Cottage cheese
Pot cheese
Farmer's cheese
Ricotta

Mozzarella
Imported Swiss
Whipped cream cheese (Temptee)
Feta, unsalted (soak covered in water to remove salt, refrigerate,
    and change water daily)
Other goat and sheep cheese (unsalted)
Whipped sweet butter
Sour cream

Raw Nuts and Seeds

Almonds (iron)
Pecans (B vitamins)
Filberts (B vitamins)
Hazelnuts (B vitamins)
Walnuts (B vitamins)
Sesame (calcium)
Pumpkin (zinc)
Sunflower (traces of all vitamins and minerals)
Pignoli, or pine nuts (vitamin E)

Fruits
(fresh, raw, or sun-dried)

Apple
Avocado
Lemon
Grapefruit (preferably with seeds)
Grapes (preferably with seeds)
Tangerine
Bosc pear
Cherries
Apricots
All melons (except cantaloupe)
Coconut (fresh only)
Kiwi (sparingly)
Currants
Peaches
Pineapple
Nectarine

Figs
Berries (all)
Mango
Papaya
Orange (sparingly)
Persimmon
Pomegranate
Lime
Banana (sparingly) (mucus-former for many people)
Dates (sparingly) (high in calcium)
Raisins (Thompson's or Monnuka)
Tomato
Black mission figs

Vegetables
(All fresh vegetables should be eaten raw, juiced, or steamed lightly)

Lettuce (any kind except iceberg)
Okra
Beets with beet tops (high in B_{12})
Parsley
Watercress
Cucumbers, preferably Kirby
Spinach (raw only; cooking releases oxalic acid, which forms kidney
    stones)
Potatoes, baked or grated raw in salad (can be eaten raw; most
    alkaline vegetable)
Yams (can be eaten raw)
Sweet potatoes (can be eaten raw)
Kale
Escarole
Chicory
Carrots with tops (if carrots are organically grown, tops may be
    used in salad)
Bok choy (Chinese cabbage/celery)
String beans
Cabbage (red preferred)
Celery
Broccoli

Zucchini
White radish
Spanish radish
Russian black radish
Dandelion greens
Jerusalem artichokes
Endive
Brussels Sprouts
Cauliflower
Swiss chard
Kohlrabi
Parsnips
Turnips
Red or green bell peppers (red are best, high in Vitamin C)
Rutabaga
Sprouts—alfalfa, mung bean, lentils, etc. (high in digestive
    enzymes)
Winter squashes, baked or steamed
Corn on the cob, lightly steamed or raw
Artichoke, steamed
Pumpkin, steamed or baked
(See Acid/Alkaline food chart for a more comprehensive list, pages
    23–24)

Oils
(cold-pressed)

Olive (extra virgin—green, crude)
Safflower
Sesame
Soy
Corn germ
Sunflower
Cold-pressed mayonnaise

Beverages

Water (distilled only)
Bottled juices (from health food store)

Fresh apple cider (which is really freshly squeezed apple juice)
Herb teas
   Comfrey leaf (healing effect)
   Rose hip (vitamin C)
   Papaya-mint (digestive aid)
   Peppermint (digestive aid)
   Spearmint (digestive aid)
   Fenugreek (helps dissolves mucus)
   Eyebright (eye antiseptic)
   Valerian root (sedative)
   Mugwort (helpful for female urinary-genital problems)
   Chamomile (digestive aid and sedative)
      NOTE: Caution must be used with herbal teas. Some can be
      harmful in improper amounts.
   Coffee substitutes
   Cafix
   Pero
   Pioneer
   Yanoh
   Blackstrap molasses (1 tsp. in 1 c. hot water is a coffee
      substitute for many)

Best Drink of All

1 fresh lemon juiced in ½–cup lukewarm or tepid water daily,
especially just before retiring. It neutralizes the system while asleep.
Be sure to rinse mouth out afterward, as it affects tooth enamel in
some people.

Best Brand-Name Products

Erewhon
Shiloh Farms
Walnut Acres
Arrowhead Mills
Hain

"No" Foods

Carbohydrates

All commercially prepared cereals and breads except those indicated
    under "Yes" Foods
White rice
Precooked oatmeal and heavily sugared dry cereals

Flours and Breads

Anything made with or containing white flour, bleached or
    unbleached
Spaghetti
Breads
Pies
Cookies
Cakes
Degerminated cornmeal

Sweeteners

Anything made with or containing white sugar
Soda pop, cooked refined honey, cane syrup
Chemical or artificial synthetic sweeteners (new ones come out
    eriodically, but all have harmful side effects)
Corn syrup
Brown sugar

Shellfish

Lobster
Shrimp
Oysters
Clams
Mussels
Crab

Preserved Meats
(contain nitrate and powerful chemical preservative that are also
mental depressants)

Salami
Bologna
Corned beef
Pastrami
Liverwurst
Hot dogs

Dairy Products

All dairy products other than those listed under ''Yes'' Foods

Nuts and Seeds

Peanuts
Brazil nuts
Cashews

Fruits

Cranberries (sparingly; okay if used with kidney, bladder, or vaginal
   infection)
Cantaloupe
Pears (Bosc pears are permissible; Bartlett and Anjou are too sweet
   for hypoglycemics and diabetics)

Oils

Mineral oil
Margarine
Lard

Seasonings

Mustard
Ketchup (permissible when purchased from health food store)
Vinegar
Pepper
MSG (monosodium glutamate)
Ginger
Curries
Baking powder containing aluminum
Table salt (small amount of sea salt is permissible)

Stimulants

Coffee
Tea
Alcohol
Ginseng

Cocoa Products

All chocolate and cocoa (hot chocolate, chocolate cake, chocolate
   candy, chocolate ice cream)

Cola Bean Products

All cola drinks

Canned and Most Frozen Foods

NOTE: Avoid all aluminum cooking utensils (aluminum has been
linked to Alzheimer's disease) and those coated with Teflon or other
synthetics. Cook foods in either enamel, stainless steel, Corning-
ware, or glass containers.

CHAPTER 7

What Are Vitamins, Anyway?

Medical researchers, including the American Cancer Society, now realize that nutrition may be the single most important factor in preventing disease and maintaining good health. The six nutrients —carbohydrates, fats, protein, vitamins, minerals, and water (plus enzymes)—are present in the foods we eat and contain chemical substances that function in one of three ways:

- They furnish the body with heat and energy.
- They provide material for growth and repair of body tissues.
- They assist in the regulation of body processes.

Each nutrient has its own specific functions and relationship to the body, but no nutrient acts independently of the others. All of the nutrients must be present in the diet in varying quantities in order for the body to maintain basic life processes. Although all of us need the same nutrients, we are all different in genetic and physiological makeup. Therefore, our quantitative nutritional needs differ.

The amount of nutrients we require is influenced by environment, level of activity, and condition of our body. Processing, storage, and preparation of food greatly affect its nutritional value.

You literally are what you eat. Optimum health, disease prevention, and longevity will be the rewards of a properly balanced diet based upon the understanding of nutrition.

Sources of Calories:
Carbohydrates, Fats, and Proteins

Carbohydrates, fats, and proteins supply fuel necessary for body heat and work, and are therefore its primary sources of energy. Their fuel potential is expressed in *calories*, a measure that determines the amount of chemical energy released as heat when foods are metabolized. Therefore, foods that are high in energy value are high in calories, while foods that are low in energy value are low in calories. Fats yield approximately nine calories per gram, and carbohydrates and proteins yield approximately four calories per gram. When you follow the nutritional regimen outlined in this book, you reach a weight that is "right" for you without counting a single calorie! How can that be, after a lifetime of calorie counting? The answer is that you satisfy your hunger with fruits and vegetables. When your meals provide you with all the nutrients your body needs, you will no longer have perverted cravings. What I teach is that when you're reasonably full and you feel good, you stop eating.

Carbohydrates

Carbohydrates are the chief source of energy for all body functions and muscular exertion. They also assist in the digestion and assimilation of other foods. Carbohydrates produce heat in the body when carbon in the system unites with oxygen in the bloodstream, providing us with immediately available calories for energy. Carbohydrates also help regulate protein and fat metabolism; fats require carbohydrates to break down within the liver.

The principal carbohydrates are sugars, starches, and cellulose. Simple sugars, such as those in honey and fruits, are very easily digested. "Double" sugars, such as refined table sugar, require some digestive action, but they are not nearly so complex as starches, such as those found in whole grains. Starches require prolonged enzymatic action in order to break them down into simple sugars (glucose) for digestion. Cellulose, commonly found in fruits and vegetables, is largely indigestible by humans and contributes little energy value to the diet. However, cellulose provides the bulk (or fiber) necessary for intestinal action and aids elimination. Diets of refined carbohydrates are usually low in vitamins, minerals, and cellulose. Such foods as white flour, white sugar, and white rice are lacking in B vitamins and other nutrients. Excessive consumption of these foods will aggravate any vitamin B deficiency an individual may have. If the B vitamins are absent, normal carbohydrate combustion cannot take place and indigestion, symptoms of heartburn, and nausea may result.

Fats

Fats, or lipids, are the most concentrated source of energy in the diet. When oxidized, fats furnish more than twice the number of calories per gram furnished by carbohydrates or proteins. One gram of fat yields approximately nine calories to the body.

In addition to providing energy, fats act as carriers for the fat-soluble vitamins, A, D, E, F, and K. By aiding in the absorption of vitamin D, fats help make calcium available to body tissues, especially to bones and teeth. Fats are also important for the conversion of carotene to vitamin A. Fat deposits surround, protect, and hold in place organs such as the kidneys, heart, and liver. Fats prolong the process of digestion by slowing down the stomach's secretions of hydrochloric acid. Thus, fats create a longer-lasting sensation of fullness after a meal.

The substances that give fats their different flavors, textures, and melting points are known as *fatty acids*. There are two types of fatty acids, saturated and unsaturated. Saturated fatty acids are those that are usually hard at room temperature and that, except for coconut oil, come primarily from animal sources. Unsaturated fatty acids, including polyunsaturates, are usually liquid at room temperature and are derived from vegetable, nut, or seed sources, such as corn, safflowers, soybeans, sunflowers, and olives. Vegetable shortenings and margarines have undergone a process called *hydrogenation*, in which unsaturated oils are converted to a more solid form of fat. Hydrogenated fats build up in the arteries and should be avoided. Other sources of fat are dairy products and eggs.

There are three "essential" fatty acids: linoleic, arachidonic, and linolenic, collectively known as unsaturated fatty acids. They are necessary for normal growth and healthy blood, arteries, and nerves. Arachidonic and linolenic acids can be synthesized from linoleic acid. These fatty acids also keep the skin and other tissues youthful and healthy, preventing dryness and scaliness. Essential fatty acids are necessary for the transport and breakdown of cholesterol.

What Is Cholesterol, and Why Are People Always Talking About It?

Cholesterol has been a cause of health and nutrition controversy for many years. It was believed that a diet high in cholesterol was the cause of atherosclerosis or narrowing of the arteries, a common element in heart conditions—the leading cause of death in this country. Now it is true that high cholesterol blood levels and atherosclerosis go hand in hand. However, it has never been satisfactorily proven that high cholesterol levels in the *diet* produce high cholesterol levels in the blood. There is considerable disagreement among authorities as to the causes of high cholesterol levels in the blood. But it is generally agreed that lack of exercise and stress are prime suspects. At the turn of the century most everybody ate high cholesterol diets, but atherosclerosis was unheard of. Why? Probably because people in general were physically active, less stressed, and the foods they ate were less refined and contaminated.

My feeling is that cholesterol counting is as unnecessary as calorie counting as long as your diet is high in raw fruits and vegetables. The cholesterol levels will then take care of themselves.

Cholesterol is essential to the body. It is a lipid or fat-related substance necessary for good health. It is a normal component of most body tissues, especially those of the brain and nervous system, liver, and blood. It is needed to form adrenal and sex hormones, vitamin D, and the bile that is needed for the digestion of fats. Cholesterol also seems to play a part in lubricating the skin. In other words, you need some cholesterol in your diet, and the case against it is overstated.

Lecithin plays an important role in maintaining a healthy nervous system, and is found naturally in the *myelin sheath*, a fatty protective covering for the nerves. Lecithin also helps to cleanse the liver and helps prevent the formation of gallstones.

Important: Avoid Rancid Oils

A certain amount of protection from rancidity is provided by vitamin E, a fat-soluble vitamin naturally present in most fatty foods. However, fats and oils should be stored in a cool place in covered containers, away from direct light, to prevent rancidity caused by oxidation. I refrigerate all my oils.

Proteins

Protein is an important factor in the maintenance of good health and vitality. It takes part in the growth of all body tissues. It is the major source of building materials for muscles, blood, skin, hair, nails, and internal organs, including the heart and the brain.

Protein is needed for the formation of hormones, which control a variety of body functions such as growth, sexual performance, and metabolic rate. It helps regulate the body's water balance. Some overzealous vegetarians cannot assimilate enough protein from vegetables or nuts and come down with edema (swelling of the ankles), and I have to get them back on some animal protein. Enzymes, substances necessary for basic life functions, and antibodies, which help fight foreign substances in the body, are also formed from protein. In addition, protein is important in the process of blood clotting and in the production of milk during lactation.

What You Should Know
About Amino Acids

The body requires twenty-two amino acids to make human protein. Twelve of these amino acids can be produced in the adult body. The ten that cannot be produced are called *essential amino acids*, and they must be supplied by the diet. Foods containing protein may or may not contain all the essential amino acids. When a food contains all the essential amino acids, it is termed *complete protein*. Foods that lack or are extremely low in any one of the essential amino acids are called *incomplete protein*. Most meats and dairy products are complete-protein foods, while most vegetables and fruits are incomplete-protein foods. To obtain a complete-protein meal from incomplete proteins, one must combine foods sensibly, so that those weak in an essential amino acid will be balanced by those strong in the same amino acid. Despite the propaganda, it is unnecessary to have complete proteins all at one time. You may consume different incomplete proteins on different days as long as they add up to complete proteins over several days.

Water

Water is the most abundant component found in the body, accounting for roughly two-thirds of body weight, and is also by far the most important nutrient. Responsible for and involved in nearly every body process, including digestion, absorption, circulation, and excretion, water is the primary transporter of nutrients throughout the body and is essential for all building functions in the body. Nearly all foods contain water that is absorbed by the body during digestion. Fruits and vegetables are especially good sources of naturally filtered pure water, which is 100 percent pure hydrogen and oxygen.

VITAMINS

Why do so many articles on vitamins tell us all about which foods we can find them in, but never what they are? Can't you tell a reader like me what a vitamin actually is and what it does? Also, why are vitamins so important and why can't vitamins be reclassified in a different way? I find the present classifications of vitamins very confusing.—Mrs. H.B.L.

I received the above letter from a reader of my newspaper column "Alive and Well" in Kingston, New York. Many people are mystified by vitamins. What is a vitamin? What does it do? In simple terms, I answered Mrs. H.B.L. (and whoever else was interested). A vitamin is an essential organic chemical substance that every living organism must obtain from its environment in minute amounts in order to survive. Vitamins play an important role in metabolism, which is a general term used to describe all the physical and chemical processes occurring within every living organism. Like any other organic substance, vitamins consist mainly of carbon, oxygen, and hydrogen in different combinations and occasionally with water, nitrogen, and phosphorus.

Certain vitamins are essential to all human beings. Some of them can be synthesized in the body; others, such as vitamin C, cannot and must be obtained from food or supplements.

A vitamin by itself is useless without a properly working enzyme. Vitamins function in tandem with chemicals called *enzymes*, which have numerous essential functions within the body. Enzymes are made up of two parts: One is a protein molecule, and the other is a coenzyme. This coenzyme is often a vitamin, or it may contain a vitamin, or it may be a molecule that has been manufactured from a vitamin. Enzymes are responsible for the oxidation process within the body. Oxygen enters the bloodstream and is transported to the cells, where oxidation actually occurs. Then the wastes are removed—carbon dioxide via the lungs and other waste products via the urine and feces. Enzymes are a major factor in biochemical processes such as growth, metabolism, cellular reproduction, and digestion. Most enzymes remain within the cells, acting as catalysts; in other words, they initiate chemical reactions that enable other materials to continue their work. Because vitamins work on the basic cellular level, a lack of one or several can cause a variety of symptoms.

Vitamins are important in our daily diet because they play an essential role in all the chemical and biological processes. Lack of vitamins can provoke many serious illnesses and may eventually result in premature death. Regarding the question about an easier vitamin classification, it is certainly far easier to refer to vitamin B_{12} than to its chemical name, cyanocobalamin, or to its chemical formula, $C_{63}H_{90}CON_{14}O_{14}P_C$, which consists of nine different substances. Perhaps someday someone will come up with a simpler terminology, but until then, let me list and describe them for you by their commonly known names.

The following will explain the function of the chief vitamins, but remember that no single vitamin should be taken in isolation from others. All nutrients work together for the good of the entire body.

Vitamin A

Vitamin A is a fat-soluble nutrient that occurs in three forms: (1) *carotene*, which is yellow in color and is found mainly in the leaves of vegetables, (2) A_1, found in the livers of saltwater fish, and (3) A_2, found in the livers of freshwater fish. A_1 and A_2 pass straight into the bloodstream and are absorbed. Carotene, from yellow, orange, and green vegetables, is acted upon by an enzyme contained in the human liver, which converts it into vitamin A. Vitamin A deficiency is not common in our society. A lack of vitamin A in the body makes absorption of vitamins difficult. A deficiency of A results in retarded growth and eye troubles such as night blindness. Vitamin A protects the body from tumors, aids in the growth and repair of the body's soft tissues, and helps maintain smooth, soft, pink, glowing, unwrinkled skin. Internally it helps protect the mucous membranes of the mouth, nose, throat, and lungs, thereby reducing susceptibility to infection, and allows the mucous membranes to combat the effects of various air pollutants. The soft tissue and all linings of the digestive tract, kidneys, and bladder are also protected by vitamin A. In addition, it promotes the secretion of gastric juices necessary for complete digestion of proteins. Another important function of vitamin A is the formation of rich blood. The American Cancer Society recommends foods rich in vitamin A and vitamin C as important elements in cancer prevention.

SOURCES: Carrots, yams, yellow squash, butter, fish liver oils, some fats, vegetable oils, pumpkin, spinach, kale, broccoli, potato, sweet potato, parsley, peas, green and red peppers, paprika, olives, peaches, apricots, and all green leafy vegetables.

Vitamin B Complex

All B vitamins are water-soluble substances. The known B-complex vitamins are B_1 (thiamine), B_2 (riboflavin), B_3 (niacin), B_5 (panthothenic acid), B_6 (pyridoxine), B_{12} (cyanocobalamin), B_{15} (pangamic acid), B_{17} (amygdalin), biotin, choline, folic acid, inositol, and PABA. The grouping of these water-soluble compounds under the blanket term *B complex* is based upon their common source, their close relationship in vegetable and animal tissues, and their functional relationships. These vitamins are active in providing the body with energy, basically by converting carbohydrates into glucose, which the body "burns" to produce energy. Processed foods are deficient in B vitamins, and a high sugar intake interferes with vitamin B assimilation. The refined diet of most Americans is usually deficient in many of the thirteen or more B vitamins.

B-complex vitamins are beneficial in treating cystitis, anemia, angina pectoris, diabetes, stroke, diarrhea, alcoholism. Deficiencies in the B's cause problems in the metabolism of fats and protein, the health of the nerves, maintenance of muscle tone in the gastrointestinal tract, and health of skin, hair, eyes, mouth, and liver.

SOURCES: Rice polish or rice bran, raw wheat germ, wheat bran, soybeans, Scottish oats, oat bran, whole rye, millet, all dark meats, chicken, kidney, liver, other whole grains and brans of every variety, all fresh and most root vegetables, avocados, most nuts and nut butter, sunflower seeds, and molasses.

Vitamin B_1 (Thiamine)

Vitamin B_1 is needed for appetite, blood building, carbohydrate metabolism, circulation, digestion, energy, growth, learning capacity, muscle tone, and maintenance of intestines, stomach, and heart. Deficiencies result in loss of appetite, digestive disturbances, fatigue, irritability, nervousness, numbness of hands and feet, pain and noise sensitivity. Excessive alcohol drains the body of vitamin B, especially B_1.

SOURCES: Blackstrap molasses, brown rice, brewer's yeast, fish, meat, nuts, poultry, and sunflower seeds.

Vitamin B$_2$ (Riboflavin)

Vitamin B$_2$ is essential for growth and is part of an enzyme mechanism through which food is burned up in the body. Frying and roasting meats destroys B$_2$; so does the boiling of milk or exposing it to strong sunlight. A deficiency is vitamin B$_2$ causes a disease known as *cheilosis* or *arboflavinosis*, characterized by a cracking and reddening of the skin at the corners of the mouth; lips and skin are abnormally red, and there is a greasy feeling at the folds between nostrils and cheeks. Sometimes patients suffering from night blindness who do not respond to vitamin A will respond to B$_2$.

> SOURCES: All plant and animal tissues, yeast, wheat germ, milk, liver, eggs, cheese, leafy vegetables, soya and other beans, avocados, lentils, and the organs of animals.

Vitamin B$_3$ (Niacin, Nicotinic Acid, Niacinamide, Nicotinamide)

Vitamin B$_3$ maintains the integrity of the mucous membrane and helps promote the normal function of the nervous system. A deficiency of niacin causes pellagra, a disease characterized by lack of pigmentation of the skin on the backs of the hands, face, and feet; inflammation of the mouth; intense soreness and redness of the tongue; neurasthenia; anxiety; dizziness; fatigue; numbness in various parts of the body (particularly the extremities); backache; headache; either constipation or diarrhea; melancholia; depression; and, in the final stages, dementia.

> SOURCES: Fresh vegetables, whole grains, brewer's yeast, liver and liver extracts, salmon, herring, cod, wheat germ, almonds, brown rice, and peanuts.

Vitamin B$_6$ (Pyridoxine)

B$_6$ is required for antibody formation, hydrochloric acid production, and fat and protein utilization, and affects the nerves through maintenance of the sodium-potassium balance. Deficiency symptoms are acne, anemia, hardening of the arteries (arteriosclerosis), arthritis, depression, and hair loss.

> SOURCES: Pecans, Blackstrap molasses, brewer's yeast, green leafy vegetables, meat, wheat germ, and whole grains.

Vitamin B$_{12}$

Vitamin B$_{12}$ is a general tonic for the body, particularly the blood and nerves. It stimulates the appetite, red blood-cell formation, and cell longevity. B$_{12}$ has been known to aid walking and speaking difficulties. The human body requires only 4 micrograms of B$_{12}$ daily, a minute dose. A deficiency of this vitamin causes fatigue, secondary anemia, and pernicious anemia.

> SOURCES: Beets and beet tops, almonds, calves' liver, nuts and seeds, dairy products, deep-sea fish (especially tuna), and eggs.

Vitamin C (Ascorbic Acid)

Vitamin C is necessary for bone and tooth formation, collagen production (the cement that holds your body together), healing burns and wounds, prevention of hemorrhaging, and resistance to colds and infectious diseases. Ascorbic acid is the most unstable of all vitamins. Heat and exposure to sunlight tend to destroy it rapidly. So does excessive cooking, pressure cooking, and the addition of bicarbonate of soda to boiled vegetables (used to preserve their color). Cooking in copper or aluminum vessels also destroys this vitamin. Citrus fruit should be eaten as soon as the skin is cut or broken, and citrus juices and milk should not be left out in strong light. A deficiency causes nosebleeds, anemia, and capillary fragility or easy bruising, and is a factor in dental decay. Even if people get enough vitamin C, its beneficial effects are cancelled out by cigarette smoking. Medical researchers find that tobacco, along with alcohol, tea, coffee, soda, antibiotics, aspirin, cortisone, stress, and high fever, destroys vitamin C in the body.

> SOURCES: Dandelions, rose hips, all citrus fruit, broccoli, berries, tomatoes, papaya, watercress, red and green peppers, all green leafy vegetables, potatoes, and strawberries.

NOTE: When you cook, you lose vitamin C. We should also use as little water as possible when cooking and make sure that lids are on tightly to prevent evaporation. Vitamin C is a very perishable vitamin and is destroyed in lengthy cooking. Any vegetable that is cooked for more than thirty minutes will lose all or most of its vitamin C value. The cooking methods used in most American homes, schools, and restaurants eliminates ninety percent or more of vitamin C. Conservation of vitamin C is especially important as surveys have shown that many American adults are deficient in this vital health substance.

Vitamin D

This vitamin is important for bone formation, heart action, nervous system maintenance, normal blood clotting, and skin respiration. A lack of vitamin D causes rickets and manifests in softening of bones and teeth. Very little vitamin D is needed for health.

SOURCES: Sunlight, egg yolks, dairy products, and liver.

Vitamin E (Tocopherol)

Vitamin E is important to the reproductive process. If women are deficient in vitamin E, it may result in barrenness and miscarriage; and in men, sterility. Vitamin E has proven effective in helping relieve phlebitis, varicose veins, muscular dystrophy, degeneration of certain parts of the eye due to advancing age, and reversing barrenness in women.

SOURCES: Dark green vegetables, avocados, all cold-pressed oils, wheat germ, most whole grains, and tomatoes.

MIRACLE MINERALS

Minerals, just like vitamins, act as catalysts for many biological reactions within the body, including muscle response, the transmission of messages through the nervous system, and digestion and metabolism of nutrients in food. They are important in the production of hormones. Minerals are absolutely essential to truly good health, especially a healthy heart. Minerals can be altered, damaged, or lost by heat in cooking. Minerals are key ingredients in your bones and are vital to the proper functioning of your nervous system. Mineral supplements will soothe frayed nerves in times of stress.

They keep nerves strong and functioning properly. A daily mineral supplement containing iron, calcium, magnesium, iodine, copper, zinc, manganese, chromium, selenium, and molybdenum can help offset an otherwise unbalanced diet. With Biochemical Reprogramming, patients are gradually weaned from mineral supplements. Young children, pregnant women, and the elderly often need extra help. The following is a list of the important minerals, with explanations of how they function in your body.

Iron

Iron is essential for the formation of hemoglobin, the part of blood that carries oxygen to the cells. It also is an active element in enzymes that help break down proteins. Deficiencies of iron cause anemia, fatigue, pallor, breathlessness, constipation, and brittle nails.

> SOURCES: Millet, beets and beet tops, kale, watercress, blackstrap molasses, beef liver, chicken liver, red meats, spinach, nuts (especially almonds), black beans, chickpeas, wheat germ.

Calcium

Calcium, vital for healthy bones and teeth, also helps regulate blood clotting, muscle function, and nerve transmission. Calcium deficiencies are responsible for muscle cramps, dental problems, and osteoporosis.

> SOURCES: Corn, millet, oatmeal, dates, all milk and dairy products, broccoli, cabbage and all leafy green vegetables, sesame seeds, molasses, kelp and dulse, and most raw nuts, especially almonds.

Magnesium

Magnesium helps the body absorb other minerals, especially calcium. Stimulates bone growth and promotes the body's use of vitamins B, C, and E. Effects of magnesium deficiency include lack of energy, muscle spasms, and weakness.

> SOURCES: Romaine lettuce, fresh raw peas, lentils, parsley, kale, spinach, escarole, and other green vegetables;

whole-grain flour and whole-meal bread, millet, and
Brazil nuts.
NOTE: Inorganic table salt (sodium chloride) impedes the assimilation of soluble calcium and magnesium. When calcium and magnesium are not properly dissolved and distributed by sodium, they
tend to form deposits in various parts of the body, obstructing
capillaries. This is one cause of gall, kidney, and bladder stones.
However, organic salt derived from fruits and vegetables (celery)
does not interfere with the metabolism of calcium and magnesium
and is especially good as a sedative for the nervous system.

Iodine

Iodine, one of the most important minerals, fuels the thyroid gland
and regulates its function. Vital for healthy skin, teeth, and nails,
iodine also promotes growth and controls energy and endurance
levels. Iodine is now recognized as an essential element for maintaining mental and physical balance. Effects of iodine deficiency
are obesity, hardening of the arteries, goiter, palpitations, irritability, dry hair, dry skin, and brittle hair and nails.
   SOURCES: Kelp, dulse, seaweeds, watercress, whole grain bread,
          yogurt, liver, and fish.

Copper

Copper combines with iron to form hemoglobin and red blood cells.
It promotes healing, protects nerve fibers, and stimulates nerve
growth. Effects of copper deficiency include chronic diarrhea, reduced resistance to disease, and nervous system damage.
   SOURCES: Apricots, currants, liver, oysters, lentils, green veg-
          etables, whole grains, almonds.

Zinc

Zinc stimulates digestion and healing. Effects of a zinc deficiency
are stunted growth, poor healing of wounds, stretchmarks, menstrual
and prostate problems, loss of taste and appetite, and sexual im-
maturity.

SOURCES: Pumpkin seeds, meat, liver, eggs, oysters, cheese, beans, lentils, whole-grain breads, cereals.

Manganese

Manganese stimulates natural enzymes, promotes bone development, and aids in production of sex hormones. Effects of manganese deficiency include deafness, dizziness, ringing in the ears, poor muscle tone, and spinal problems.

SOURCES: Watercress, whole-grain cereals, egg yolks, green vegetables, nuts, seeds.

Chromium

Affects blood sugar level and glucose metabolism (energy). Helps diabetes. Effects of chromium deficiency include fatigue, lack of energy, and indigestion.

SOURCES: Minute amounts in many whole-grain cereals, particularly corn, and fresh fruits and vegetables.

Selenium

Combines with vitamin E to promote fertility, is thought to protect against cancer, and improves condition of arteries. Effects of selenium deficiency are premature aging, eye and nerve disorders, and infertility.

SOURCES: Millet, meat, fish, dairy products, raw grains, and brewer's yeast.

Potassium

Potassium, an essential mineral lacking in many diets, helps build and support the entire muscular system. If it is missing in the diet, the heart valves may shrink, resulting in blood regurgitation (heart murmur). Potassium is necessary to keep blood and tissues slightly alkaline. Sufficient potassium is essential for healing injuries, cuts, and bruises, promoting the proper functioning of the nervous system and improving nerve conductivity, muscular coordination, and hair health. It is essential for growth, stimulates nerve impulses, promotes healthy skin, helps process sugars, boosts kidney function, aids in the elimination of body wastes, and combines with sodium to regulate heartbeat. Effects of potassium deficiency include insomnia, irregular heartbeat, constipation, acne, dry skin, sagging muscles, and nervous disorders. A lack of this important mineral may lead to periodic throbbing headaches, lusterless eyes and poor eyesight, abnormal perspiration, muscular atrophy, numbness, fever, ulcers and other stomach ailments, digestive disturbances, and prolapsus of the stomach, kidneys, bladder, uterus. Results in muscle spasms and loss of muscle tone.

> SOURCES: Apples, avocados, watermelon, banana, oranges, baked potatoes, romaine lettuce, spinach and other leafy green vegetables, millet, barley, oats, brown rice and other whole grains, and sunflower seeds. (The vegetables highest in potassium are zucchini, yellow squash, potatoes, watercress, parsley, and carrots.)

Phosphorus

Phosphorus is an important mineral for bone and brain and is necessary for the nutrition of various nerve centers in the body. Phosphorus ensures proper growth and repair of cells and the growth of bones and teeth. It helps digest proteins, fats, and carbohydrates. It has a direct effect upon blood production. Phosphorus deficiency results in soft bones, atrophy of the brain cells, poor growth, problems with teeth and bones, arthritis, fatigue, and loss of appetite.

> SOURCES: Meat, poultry, eggs, fish, whole grains, seeds, and nuts.

Fluoride

A distinction should be made between calcium fluoride and sodium fluoride. Calcium fluoride strengthens bones, protects against tooth decay. A deficiency provokes tooth decay and tooth loss. Sodium fluoride, a rat poison and a harmful inorganic mineral (a by-product of the manufacture of aluminum industry) is now added to many city water supplies ostensibly to prevent cavities.

SOURCES: All seafoods, meat, cheese, nuts and seeds, millet.

VITAMINS, MINERALS, AND THE MEANING OF NUTRITION

Proper nutrition means that all the essential nutrients—carbohydrates, fats, protein, vitamins, minerals, and water—are supplied and utilized in adequate balance to maintain optimal health and well-being. Nutritional deficiencies result whenever inadequate amounts of essential nutrients are provided to tissues that must function normally over a long period of time. Good nutrition is essential for normal organ development and function; for normal reproduction, growth, and maintenance; for optimal activity level and working efficiency; for resistance to infection and disease; and for the ability to repair bodily damage or injury.

No single food, vitamin, or mineral will ensure or maintain vibrant health. Although specific nutrients are known to be more important in the functioning of certain parts of the body, even these depend upon the presence of other nutrients to function properly. Every effort should therefore be made to attain and maintain a balanced daily intake of all the necessary nutrients throughout life. Assimilation is what counts. You can eat the most wonderful food in the world, organically grown and expensive, but if your body, *your specific body*, cannot absorb and utilize that food, you will eventually suffer from nutritional deficiencies and ill health.

Certainly, *beyond the shadow of a doubt*, the foundation of all health is nutrition, and the secret of good nutrition is a diet consisting mainly of fruits and vegetables.

CHAPTER 8

Secrets of Raw Fruits and Vegetables

Consumption of fresh vegetables has grown 12 percent since 1980, according to the Agriculture Department. . . . More Americans are adopting some of the principles of vegetarianism and may even proclaim themselves to be vegetarians, associating a diet of vegetables, beans and grains with wholesomeness, healthfulness and nutritional enlightenment. . . . Despite the increased interest in vegetarian options, the country still clings to its carnivorous habits. In 1985, according to the Agriculture Department, Americans ate more animal flesh than ever: 237.4 pounds per capita of red meat, chicken and fish, up more than six pounds from 1980.

—The New York Times, March 25, 1987

Those of you who cling to your "carnivorous habits," either because of a preference for meat or a concern about "enough protein," should realize by now that a predominantly vegetarian diet is nutritionally superior to a diet high in animal protein. You don't need lots of proteins from meat, fowl, and fish. Propaganda that says you do is just that, propaganda! Vegetable sources—lentils, chick-peas, soybeans, millet, brown rice, and whole grains—provide protein in abundance. With a little ingenuity, you can prepare hundreds of exciting, palatable, nutritious, and economical meals, using combinations of my twenty favorite "superfoods" (see recipes, chapter 6).

TWENTY SUPER FOODS

1. Apples

Although it may not be absolutely factual to say that "an apple a day keeps the doctor away," this fruit certainly can help keep many health problems at bay and improve others (depending on one's digestive abilities). Apples contain proteins, carbohydrates, some fat, minerals, some calories, and vitamins A, B, and C. Apples are rich in vitamin C, so they are especially beneficial for those subject to frequent colds (keeping the doctor away). They help prevent gingivitis (bleeding gums). Apples are one of the richest sources of potassium, essential for healing.

Ideally, apples should be eaten raw. Unfortunately, apples today are sprayed with chemicals that adhere to the skin of the apple, though some may be removed with a vinegar bath. But why eat poison if you don't have to? Peel off the skin.

The B vitamins in apples help certain nerve disorders. The iron counteracts the tendency toward anemia and aids in the formation of red blood cells. Apples nourish bone and muscle. Since the normal American diet usually contains excess salt, the sodium and potassium in apples will help flush it out of the system.

Since they contain about 84 percent water, apples are a good source of daily fluid intake. When you're thirsty, an apple is far more health-giving and thirst-quenching than is water, coffee, tea, soda, or, in the summer, iced drinks. As thirst-slakers, fresh raw fruits are far superior to the constant drinking of water and other liquids.

Malic acid, in which apples are rich, dissolves and flushes out wastes from the body, particularly cellulite deposits.

An apple or two chewed slowly and thoroughly before retiring helps bring on normal bowel action in the morning and also, strangely enough, helps stop diarrhea. Eat only peeled apples, or baked apples without skins, for two or three days, until all traces of diarrhea are gone.

Note: Don't eat apples if you have gallbladder problems, often signaled by a pain under the right side after eating.

2. Avocados

There are 17 vitamins and minerals present in the creamy, yellow or greenish flesh of this nutritious semi-tropical fruit. Avocados are rich in vitamins A and C and contain significant amounts of vitamins B_1, B_2, B_3 and E. Minerals include phosphorous, magnesium, sodium, calcium, iron, zinc, copper, and manganese. The ratio of very high potassium to very low sodium provides an excellent nutritional balance. (The avocado's level of potassium exceeds that of bananas!) Avocados are an ideal fruit because they are "nutrient dense": There is a high return of nutrients to calorie intake.

The amount of oil in an avocado varies seasonally, but the average is about 16%. Most of this is in the form of easy-to-digest, natural monounsaturated fatty acids. According to one body of medical opinion, this prevents cholesterol from being deposited in the blood vessels, tending to reduce the risk of heart attacks and hardening of the arteries.

When I tell my patients this, many say, "But Dr. Soltanoff, I thought avocados were high in cholesterol." In fact, this superfruit of nature contains absolutely NO CHOLESTEROL, and I recommend it for people who must watch their cholesterol intake. (See recipe section)

Avocados have a rich flavor and are easily digestible, combining well in your daily diet with other fruits and vegetables. There are three 'races' of avocados—Mexican, Guatemalan, and West Indian. The avocados most commonly available in the U.S. are the Guatemalan and hybrids of the Guatemalan and Mexican races. Today, due to their increasing popularity, avocados are grown in semi-tropical countries throughout the world. Many of our best avocados are grown in California and Florida . . . I prefer the California variety for its rich nutty flavor. For the 76% of us who are concerned about the danger of pesticides, a very important advantage of avocados is that they are rarely chemically sprayed.

Avocados are eaten raw. Ripe avocados that are not eaten immediately should be refrigerated; they'll last several days. If I don't use the whole avocado, I store the rest in the refrigerator with skin and pit intact, sealed in plastic wrap. (See recipe section)

3. Broccoli

Broccoli is the only vegetable that contains traces of all the nutrients. It is especially rich in vitamins A and C, calcium, and potassium. Broccoli and the other vegetables in its family—cabbage, Brussels sprouts, kohlrabi, and cauliflower—are thought to provide protection against the development of some cancers. The word on broccoli is out. Broccoli consumption is up 767 percent over the last twenty years. (See recipe section)

4. Cabbage

Cabbage is a marvelous vegetable high in vitamin C. It is also rich in choline, which is part of the vitamin B complex, which nourishes the muscular system. Lack of choline is a factor in narrowed and hardened arteries and other serious ailments. In addition to vitamins B and C, cabbage contains traces of iron and iodine—also found in abundance in onions, sprouts, watercress, spinach, and carrots. The cellulose in cabbage provides relief from constipation. Red cabbage has more nutrients than white cabbage and is therefore more valuable. Chinese cabbage and bok choy are less sprayed and more easily assimilated than regular cabbage. (See recipe section) There are indications that cabbage is a factor in muscle strength and in promoting endurance.

5. Carrots

Carrots are noted for their high vitamin A content. A small carrot, eaten raw after a meal, cleanses the tooth enamel and helps prevent cavities. Carrots provide potent health-building materials, owing to outstanding amounts of vitamin A compounds (essential for good eyesight) together with iodine, iron, and copper and vitamin E. (See recipe section) Perhaps even more important, beta carotene (with which carrots are richly endowed) is becoming recognized as a powerful cancer preventative. While masses of vitamin A supplements can be toxic, only good can come from eating more carrots.

6. Corn

Corn is a very rich source of calcium phosphate. I highly recommend it as a calcium source over milk and other dairy products. My wife and I once drove to an isolated little Indian village in Mexico where the natives ate only corn bread, corn soup, raw corn on the cob, and corn everything else. They had the most marvelous physiques of any people I had ever seen. They were straight, tall, and strong, with wonderfully white teeth. One day a woman came from the neighboring village twenty-seven miles away to tell our landlady that her sister, who lived in this village, had become seriously ill. No one was taking care of her or the children. Our landlady, a very organized, intelligent woman, immediately got herself ready. She arose at 3:00 A.M., and walked, jogged, and ran the twenty-seven miles to the village where her sister lived. There she found friends and neighbors to take care of the sister and her children and then walked, jogged, and ran the twenty-seven miles back the same day. If the average American jogger in Central Park ran fifty-four miles a day, he or she would be carried away in a casket. That woman and the people in her village lived on a simple diet composed of a few fruits and a great deal of vegetables, predominantly corn. I am convinced this simplicity and the emphasis on vegetables, rather than a diet high in dairy-based calcium, was responsible for their overall vitality.

You can eat raw or lightly steamed corn on the cob for breakfast. There is considerable protein in corn. In the summertime I take a break from the baked potatoes and millet that I love most of the year and three or four days a week eat a high-protein and calcium dinner of two ears of corn with a big salad. I know it sounds peculiar—raw corn! But try it, it's delicious.

7. Lemons

Today the invincible lemon is cultivated in many different countries and is obtainable year-round, but it was unknown to our distant ancestors. Native to India, the lemon was introduced into Spain by Arabs in the twelfth century, but it was not until around 1500 that lemon plantations became firmly established in both Spain and Portugal.

Lemons played an important role in the prevention and elimination of scurvy, which commonly afflicted sailors in the days of the old sailing ships. Scurvy, a debilitating condition characterized by spongy, bleeding gums, loosening of teeth, and total loss of energy, produced more fatalities than storms and shipwreck. One of the early pioneers in the medical field of prevention was a Scottish physician, James Lind. On his advice the British Admiralty prescribed the use of lime or lemon juice for the specific prevention of scurvy. As a consequence, scurvy was wiped out almost overnight, and English sailors became known as limeys.

No other fruit has such a great variety of uses, and no other fruit in the citrus group, or in any other group, can compare with the lemon in its valuable properties internally and externally as an antiseptic purifier, cleanser, and neutralizer. Following are some of the properties and uses of the lemon, which have been developed in many different countries over the years:

NOTE: Lemons are not indicated for those suffering from ulcers.

• *To relieve heartburn and indigestion:* Lemon tastes acid, but in fact it neutralizes other acids, as it is highly alkaline-producing. Half a medium lemon squeezed into an eight-ounce glass of lukewarm or tepid water and slowly sipped gives quick relief from symptoms of indigestion. Try it instead of an antacid.

• *To cure a hangover:* The juice of two lemons in a glass of warm water should be repeated hourly until all hangover symptoms are gone. It works like a charm! The booze highly acidifies your body and the lemon swiftly redresses the balance.

• *To cleanse the hands after preparing food:* Rub a cut lemon on hands to bleach out stains and neutralize food odors.

• *To disinfect cuts and wounds:* Apply undiluted fresh lemon juice several times a day. It stings, but it heals in a hurry.

• *To soothe aches and pains:* Add the juice of one lemon to warm olive oil, then massage.

• *To enhance and improve the flavor of many dishes:* A final squirt of lemon will bring out the natural flavors.

• *To make pastries lighter and tastier:* Add the juice of one lemon to pies and cookies (if bake you must).

• *To remove stains from laundry:* After soaping, add to final rinse water.

• *For overall health:* One-half a medium lemon squeezed into one-half glass of lukewarm or tepid water just before retiring has a remarkable sedative effect on your nervous system. Work up to one whole lemon. (Do not use bottled concentrate.) It alkalizes and helps your body heal as you sleep, with nothing else interfering in the process. You will wake up more refreshed and revitalized. (Be sure to rinse your mouth out afterward with plain water and swish the water around to wash the lemon juice off the teeth or brush your teeth, since over time it can eat away tooth enamel.)

8. Millet

Seven reasons to make millet the predominant grain of your daily diet:

1. It is the only alkaline grain.
2. It is nonfattening.
3. It is easily digested.
4. It has a mild laxative effect.
5. It is so versatile that many dishes can be made from it or enhanced by it.
6. It is the only protein grain.
7. It tastes great raw or cooked.

Millet has all the essential amino acids and is particularly rich in the B vitamins riboflavin and thiamine. It also contains substantial quantities of vitamins A and C. It has more minerals than other grains and is rich in potassium, sodium, calcium, magnesium, iron, and fluorine. Millet has been used in Europe, Asia, and Africa as a remedy for colitis and stomach ulcers and to help kidney, bladder, and urinary complaints.

The name "millet" is derived through the Italian from the Latin word for "thousand," because of the tiny, round, seed-pearl sized grains. You can live for long periods on millet alone and still stay healthy, but I wouldn't want to do it out of choice.

Millet dates back to prehistoric times and may have been the first grain cultivated by humans when hunting gave way to husbandry and agriculture. Archaeologists discovered evidence of its early cultivation in the remains of early lake-dweller settlements in Switzerland as well as in ancient Egyptian tombs. It was an important staple food in biblical times and considered sacred by the Chinese as far back as 2500 B.C. Pythagoras, the ancient vegetarian Greek philosopher, urged all his followers to eat millet to improve their health and strength. Attila, king of the Huns, fed all important visitors, including royalty and ambassadors, almost exclusively with this grain.

Millet is grown chiefly in the southeast regions of the USSR and in America, Asia, and Africa. Millet is commonly ground into flour, cooked as a whole grain, and frequently eaten raw. (Sprinkle a spoonful of raw millet over your salad for instant health crunch.)

Recent experiments at Yale University have shown that millet is richer in protein, vitamins, minerals, and unsaturated fat than any other grain. Apart from its essential amino acids, millet also provides a considerable amount of lecithin, which in turn furnishes the important B vitamin choline, which helps keep cholesterol fluid. As long as cholesterol remains fluid, the formation of certain types of gallstones, hardening of the arteries, thrombosis, and other ailments caused by cholesterol buildup are unlikely.

Millet flakes and puffed millet, which can be purchased in health food stores, are an excellent breakfast with hot or cold apple juice added.

9. Nuts

Nuts are a concentrated food source of proteins, unsaturated fats, the B-complex vitamins, vitamin E, calcium, iron, potassium, magnesium, phosphorus, and copper. They should be eaten raw (not roasted) or ground into butter (always unsalted). Nuts may interfere with digestion unless they are chewed well or chopped fine.

If you think of nuts as just a premeal appetizer you should do some rethinking. Knowledgeable vegetarians know how versatile nuts are and how valuable as sources of unsaturated oils, proteins, vitamins, and minerals. A gourmet will tell you that nuts add style, character, and delicious new flavors to dishes as different as chicken and ice cream.

Some medical nutritionists and dieticians (who should know better) still talk about nuts as second-class protein because they lack two essential amino acids. But these two missing proteins are present in so many other foods (green vegetables, legumes, eggs, and dairy products) that unless you eat nothing but nuts, any of these foods will supply the necessary proteins.

You would find it very difficult to put together any kind of meat dish that comes close in value to a small dish of nuts. Many nuts are 50 percent oil. (When you leave some chopped nuts on a paper napkin for a few minutes, the oil stains the paper.) Nut oil is high in polyunsaturated fatty acids and vitamin E, which keep your brain and nervous system at maximum efficiency. Fortunately, because of their high calorie count, you don't have to eat many nuts to get a meal's worth of energy and valuable nutrition. This means also that nuts are not quite as expensive as they seem. You are buying a very concentrated food.

Nuts in their shells are freshest and best. You can keep them in your refrigerator for months in airtight jars or cans. If you buy shelled nuts, buy whole ones rather than the chopped or broken varieties, which become rancid quickly. Even whole, shelled almonds, walnuts, and pecans won't keep fresh for more than three or four months. The warmer the weather and the hotter the storage place, the more rapidly they become rancid. So always keep them in your refrigerator. Shelled nuts have already been dried to some extent. You can freshen them and pick up their flavor by soaking them in water for twenty-four to forty-eight hours, as you would dried fruit.

My favorite nut—the only alkaline nut rich in iron, calcium, and potassium—is the almond. Most almonds are grown in the United States. Edgar Cayce, the clairvoyant healer, believed that five or six almonds a day could neutralize an incipient cancer in the body.

International law says nuts must be fumigated before they're loaded onto cargo ships. Then, after a certain amount of time, they must be fumigated again. Cashews coming from India are fumigated a second time near Gibraltar. The United States will not let cashews into this country unless they're fumigated a third time. Thus imported cashews, fumigated three times, are the most contaminated nuts available. Cashews are one of the most acid-forming nuts.

10. Oatmeal

Oats are one of the most nutritious of all the cereals. Analysis places them high on the list of body-building foods. They keep tissues and nerves in healthy condition and help neutralize excess cholesterol. Oatmeal's protein content is easily absorbed and assimilated. Oats contain less starch or carbohydrate than most cereals and contain more calcium, phosphorus, and iron. They are also rich in the B vitamins riboflavin, thiamine, and niacin. Vitamin E is also present, and oats are a good source of iodine. However, oats are one of the most acidic of cereals and among the highest in gluten content. Therefore, eat them sparingly. On a cold, bone-chilling winter day, there is nothing like a bowl of hot oatmeal.

11. Papaya

Papayas are tropical fruits with fleshy, peach-colored interiors studded with dozens of black seeds. Cut the fruit in half and you can easily scoop out the seeds. The flesh is sweet and rich in digestive enzymes and vitamin C. (Twenty-two years ago my wife and I went to a Mexican spa filled with people seriously sick with leg sores, ulcers, diabetes, and other ailments. A medical doctor, more experimental than most, put these people on a diet of sliced papaya alone and distilled water three or four times a day for a month. Papaya contains a substance called *papain*, reputed to have healing properties. It breaks down foreign substances in the body, including uric and other toxic acids. I observed that many of the ailments, particularly the ulcers, were healed or helped by the exclusive papaya regimen.)

12. Parsley

Parsley is a valuable high-potency herb with a concentrated vitamin A and C content. The ancients knew that parsley had medicinal value and used every part of the plant—leaves, stems, roots, and seeds—for kidney and skin disorders. Parsley is particularly useful because of its concentrated nature. A handful of parsley chewed raw is a superior breath freshener.

13. Parsnips

Parsnips are high in vitamins A and B and phosphorus, the mineral necessary for the health of bones, brain, and muscular tissue. Parsnips are an antiflatulant and are highly alkaline-forming and easy to digest. (See recipes, page 000.)

14. Potatoes

Among the reasons the Irish took to the potato was that it was easily grown in their country, hardier than wheat or barley, and occupied less space for an equivalent yield. In rural areas, the economy is still based on the potato. The cuisine includes potato bread, potato pancakes, and potato soup. One of the longest-lived people in the Western world are the rural Irish. The potato, alkaline-producing and rich in protein, minerals, and vitamins, is an almost perfect food. (Potato experimenters have lived for up to three hundred days on potatoes and a little fat.) Depending upon their freshness, potatoes consist of 80 percent water, 3.7 percent protein, and about 16 percent carbohydrates in the form of easily assimilated starch. They are high in potassium and vitamins A, B, and C.

People don't get tired of potatoes. A baked potato and salad dinner becomes the mainstay of my patients' diets and remains so after they are restored to health. I eat a potato/salad dinner about four times a week. It's the perfect, easy-to-prepare meal in a fast-paced society.

15. Sea Products and Sea Plants

The oceans contain many nourishing substances high in protein, minerals, and vitamins. Marine biologists say a seaweed crop taken from the Atlantic Ocean alone would amount to more than 20,000 times the entire world's annual grain harvest. Nutritionists strongly recommend the liberal use of dulse, kelp, and other sea products in our daily diet. Apart from plants, the oceans provide valuable fish oil products from cod, halibut, and herring.

Food manufacturers in the United States, Canada, Norway, Morocco, South America, South Africa, Sweden, and Denmark now make large quantities of fish flour for human consumption from fish and fish by-products. The manufacture of this fish concentrate is strongly backed by fisheries and nutritionists associated with the World Food and Health Organization, who hope that this may be the means of feeding undernourished millions all over the world. Its protein content amounts to a very high 75 to 80 percent.

Let us take a closer look at the health properties of seaweed. All varieties are rich in important minerals, vitamins, and protein compounds.

Seaweed is unusually high in protein and contains all forty-three trace minerals. The iodine in seaweed stimulates the thyroid and parathyroid glands so they can better absorb the calcium that seaweed provides, nourishing bones and joints. I crumble a thin sheet of crisp nori seaweed into my salad daily.

Seaweed can help specific disorders such as the following:

Arthritis. This condition is sometimes caused by calcium and mineral imbalance. Joints harden, bones become brittle, sufferers have cold hands and feet. The minerals in seaweed, especially iodine, speed up metabolism for better mineral absorption.

Osteoporosis (brittle bones). Seaweed contains calcium phosphate, a mineral that strengthens bones, thereby helping prevent osteoporosis and other bone-related problems.

PMS and nosebleeds. Calcium deficiency, often associated with PMS and nosebleeds, may be alleviated by eating seaweed. Daily portions of seaweed will furnish the calcium needed to forestall these painful and frightening episodes.

Cancer. Many medical researchers now believe cancer results from a combination of food, drink, lifestyle habits, genetics, and pollutants. Nutritionists believe that the calcium, iodine, and sodium alginate in seaweed could well serve as a buffer against cancer, since their preventative effect in other diseases is well-attested.

Seaweed is also rich in potassium, which nourishes the heart and kidneys. Potassium is an essential element in almost all healing processes. While losing weight may not be a prime reason for eating seaweed, it is a factor in slimming. Its high iodine content helps regulate the thyroid gland, which in turn controls energy level, weight loss and gain. Seaweed also helps maintain the health of the mucous membrane and is a valuable adjunct to the treatment of arthritis, constipation, nervous disorders, colds, and skin irritations.

The most common forms of seaweed, dulse and kelp, are available in health food stores and Oriental markets. Both can be cooked and served like spinach. Dulse and kelp powder can be used as a seasoning.

Kelp is a common species of seaweed found in all oceans and is especially abundant along the Irish and Scottish coasts. It contains at least sixteen different minerals, including calcium, potassium, sodium, silicon, zinc, selenium, barium, and chromium. Vitamins A, B, D, and E are also found in kelp, which also comes in tablet form. (Kelp powder, which looks like pepper and tastes like salt, can be used as a seasoning or salt substitute. This is a good example of substituting something beneficial to one's health for something harmful. As we know, table salt is a nerve and heart irritant and is harmful to the kidneys.)

Another edible seaweed, sea dulse, is the most nutritious of all seaweeds. It is harvested off the shores of Nova Scotia and California. All forty-three trace minerals are found in dulse. Eating both dulse and kelp together will give you your daily quota of minerals—inexpensively.

16. Seeds

Pumpkin seeds, sesame seeds, and sunflower seeds are rich in protein, the B complex, vitamins A, D, and E, phosphorus, calcium, iron, fluorine, iodine, potassium, magnesium, zinc, and unsaturated fatty acids. Whole hulled sesame seeds are more than fifty percent calcium—another excellent substitute for mucous-forming dairy products.

17. Soybeans

The soybean, king of all beans, is the most important of all the 150-odd species of bean known. The Chinese considered the soybean vital to civilization and included it among their five essential sacred foods, along with barley, millet, rice, and wheat.

Oriental cultures sprouted soybeans, made soy milk, soybean "cheese," curd, and sauce from them. Virtually unknown in the United States or Europe until about 1900, the soybean is now playing an ever-increasing role as a cereal, oil, margarine, flour, and milk substitute.

Soybeans have a protein content equal to meat, fish, or fowl —so the wise ancient Chinese thousands of years ago were justified in calling the soybean "the meat of the soil."

Soybeans contain 40 percent protein and 18 percent unsaturated vegetable fat. It is one of the foods along with millet, sunflower seeds, and animal protein to contain all the amino acids. Soybeans also contain vitamins A, B, E, thiamine, niacin, and riboflavin, and the minerals copper, iron, and calcium.

All soy products are rich sources of lecithin, which is found in comparatively few foods. (Other sources are egg whites and raw wheat germ, which I generally do not recommend.) I can't overstress the importance of lecithin. Lecithin is utilized by the body to strengthen the nervous system. It contains two important substances, choline and inositol, which counteract the buildup of fatty deposits in the body.

Soybeans, an inexpensive and satisfying element in the quest for health, are also available in the form of soy milk, a tasty and nutritious substitute for cow's milk. Use it in cereals, cooking, and baking. If you are going to play hookey by drinking coffee, use soy milk instead of cream.

18. Tomato

There are certain nutritional schools who outlaw the tomato, a member of the nightshade family (along with potatoes and belladonna). I feel this is a mistake. To me, the tomato is one of the most valuable foods. The sweetest tomatoes, richest in vitamin C, are local and organically grown, fresh-picked and ripe. When local tomatoes are out of season, buy cherry tomatoes or Italian plum tomatoes.

Tomatoes consist of 94 percent water, .9 percent protein, .2 percent fat, 3.75 percent carbohydrates, and 1.28 percent mineral matter, mainly potassium, phosphorus, calcium, and sulfur. In addition to vitamin C, tomatoes contain vitamins A and K.

A few tomatoes with an animal-protein meal help neutralize uric acid and contribute to digestion. Tomato juice is a healthful drink. But if you buy it instead of making it yourself, be sure it is not loaded with salt. Unsalted tomato juice is usually available in health food stores.

19. Watercress

Watercress is a major green and deserves to be considered as a food instead of as a garnish. An aquatic salad plant and, suprisingly, a member of the cabbage family, watercress is rich in minerals, particularly manganese, which helps to nourish the pituitary gland and strengthen the spine. It also contains copper, magnesium, sodium, potassium, considerable calcium, and iron. Only dulse and kelp contain more iron. Watercress is therefore good for those with anemic conditions. The sulfur in watercress helps regulate the endocrine system and has an especially beneficial effect on the pancreas. This high sulfur content gives watercress its peppery taste, which stimulates the appetite and peps up bland foods so that the usual harmful condiments—salt, pepper, mustard, and vinegar—are unnecessary. It is also an important source of iodine. Medical authorities agree that a lack of iodine leads to a variety of ailments, including thyroid problems, arthritis, anemia, mental and emotional problems, and a general slowdown of activity and stamina. I like to munch on a few stalks of watercress while I am preparing my dinner.

20. Yogurt

Being practical, I know how difficult it is for people to give up or even drastically curtail dairy products. Yogurt is a dairy product, but with many good points in its favor. Yogurt is okay as long as you do not eat more than four ounces a day, especially if you also eat animal protein. Yogurt helps neutralize uric acid. But for vegetarians, yogurt is unnecessary. Goat's and mare's milk were originally used in making yogurt. Both are greatly superior to cow's milk; they are richer in nutrients and easier to digest. Unfortunately, whenever the public recognizes the value of a natural food, synthetic imitations instantly appear to fill the demand. So it is with yogurt. Valueless commercial starters are now used by many in making cow's milk "yogurt," with a milk curd and a flavor designed to imitate true goat's milk yogurt. But this commercial yogurt lacks many of the beneficial organisms and enzymes found in goat's milk yogurt. There are, however, cow's milk yogurts—Columbo, Brown Cow, Lacto, and Continental, for example—that use good starters and produce a superior product.

It is easy to make yogurt at home using certified raw milk or goat's milk and an inexpensive incubator or starter kit. Eat only plain yogurt, adding your own fresh fruit.

When yogurt cools after processing, its two types of beneficial enzymes go dormant. However, when this yogurt is eaten and reaches body heat of 98.6, these digestive enzymes are reactivated. This allows the enzymes and digestive juices to penetrate deeply into the foods in the digestive tract. This process continues in the bowels, resulting in soft and malleable feces and easier, more complete bowel movements.

Yogurt contains enzymes that suppress the putrefactive organisms in incompletely digested food. This prevents "gas" and that "full" feeling after meals. (Elderly people with insufficient digestive enzymes—a condition prevalent today among the young as well—will find yogurt especially beneficial.)

Progressive medical doctors have been prescribing yogurt for patients whose intestinal flora and fauna have been weakened or damaged by treatment with sulfa drugs or antibiotics. It is a fact that the Balkan countries, where people eat natural goat's milk yogurt daily with every meal, boast one of the highest per capita percentages of centenarians in the world. People there are famous for their clear skins, almost indestructible teeth, and absence of intestinal problems.

STORING, CLEANING, AND COOKING FRUITS AND VEGETABLES

Storing Fruits and Vegetables

It is best to wash fresh fruits and vegetables just before using. If you wash them before storing to save time, drain thoroughly to remove moisture, which speeds deterioration.

Vegetables should always be stored separately from fruits because they give off different gases. Overexposure to air and warm temperatures robs them of vitamins.

Store potatoes and onions in a cool, dry, dark place or in your refrigerator to prevent sprouting. Hard-rind squash, rutabaga, and sweet potatoes should be stored at about 60 degrees or in your refrigerator.

Cleaning Fruits and Vegetables

Do not soak fruits and vegetables in water for long periods. Water-soluble vitamins will leach out.

Wash fruits and vegetables in white vinegar (acetic acid) to rid them of most of the petroleum-oil-based insecticides—poison to the human body. Use two tablespoons of white vinegar to a gallon of tap water and let your fruits and vegetables soak for about 5 minutes. Rinse and dry. This will get rid of at least some of the surface sprays.

Scrub vegetables with edible skins, such as potatoes, rather than peeling them, to save all the fiber.

Cooking Fruits and Vegetables

Eat the outer, nutrient-rich leaves as well as the inner leaves of cabbage and lettuce.

Vitamin C, the B vitamins, and some mineral salts and iron are water-soluble and wash out of food when boiled. To minimize this loss, cut vegetables into large pieces or leave them whole and steam them or cook in as little water as possible. Of course, to steam foods that have to cook longer, such as potatoes or beets, you would use more water. Steaming is a great way to cook vegetables because it uses little water. Don't overcook. Never add baking soda to the cooking liquid of vegetables. Soda destroys thiamine and vitamin C.

When you sauté vegetables, use a minimum amount of a good oil like cold-pressed sesame oil or virgin olive oil. Have a great big salad along with it. Most people who eat sautéed and fatty foods also eat lots of cooked foods with them. If you don't have a salad in conjunction with your cooked or sautéed vegetables, you will get a buildup of mineral deposits or plaque in your body. Plaque comes from cooked foods, not just from fats and dairy products. I must stress time and again that between 60 and 70 percent of your diet should be fresh fruits and vegetables in proper combinations. If you pay attention to this, you don't have to be too concerned about the rest.

What About Frozen and Canned Vegetables?

Frozen vegetables are not as good as fresh vegetables, but not as bad as canned, precooked vegetables. To freeze vegetables manufacturers parboil them, and vitamins and minerals are lost. But they have not been cooked to death as in canning. Freezing is a far better method than canning where there is such a close relationship between the food and the can that the food takes on some of the properties of the container.

The Importance of Eating Locally Grown Foods

It is important to eat locally grown foods. Foods transported across the country lose many nutrients in transit. Who knows how long they've been in transport and storage! Local foods are fresher, crisper, and will be freer from preservative spray. In general, mass-produced, commercially grown vegetables are heavily dosed with pesticides and preservative chemicals. Imported foods are even worse. Many are sprayed with lethal chemicals banned in the United States. Regulations generally flaunted in the United States do not even exist in many thirdworld countries. According to the General Accounting Office, less than 1 percent of all imported produce is checked for traces of illegal pesticides.

Obviously, fruits and vegetables that you grow yourself organically are the best. It is no accident that gardening is America's number one hobby today. Next best are local farmers' markets and stands. Americans are wising up—in a recent survey 76 percent believed that pesticides and herbicides continue to pose a major threat to food supplies.

CHAPTER 9

The Bitter Truth About the Foods You Love

There are many foods that should be cut out or curtailed in the pursuit of health, and some of these are staples in practically everyone's diet. They range from bad to worse to poison. But I am a realist. Not many of us are desert monks. If your health is very good, or even just pretty good, and you really crave that drink, slice of Black Forest cake, morning coffee, or filet mignon, an occasional indulgence is not going to do you any harm. Moderation is the key. Let's look at these foods, and why I think they should be avoided or eaten cautiously, starting with the most harmful.

1. ANIMAL PROTEIN

I know how difficult it is to cut down on meat. But there is not much good to be said about meat—and even less good to be said about today's intensively raised, chemical-laced, and hormone-injected meat. (There are 20,000 animal drugs in use. Of these, only 10 percent have been approved under the formal FDA process.)

Animal foods are relatively easily digested, more so than vegetable sources of protein such as beans, lentils, nuts, and seeds.

212

However, animal products start to putrefy one-quarter of the way down the intestinal tract. Uric acid and many other toxins are produced that the body cannot easily assimilate or totally excrete. Over a period of time this often results in gout, rheumatism, arthritis, cysts and tumors, premature aging, and general disease. Yes, yes, I know about your uncle Joe who lived to be ninety-seven and had bacon and eggs for breakfast and a two-pound steak for supper every day of his life. But what about all those young people with hardening of the arteries and heart attacks while still in their twenties? There is no doubt in the minds of many orthodox medical researchers that overconsumption of animal protein is a major player in America's ill health.

What About Chicken and Fish?

Those who've become suspicious of red meat and switched over to chicken and fish are deluding themselves. Patients come to me and tell me they've given up red meat and they're eating only chicken and fish, and they think I should pin a medal on them, I tell them there is nothing wrong with red meat that is not also wrong with chicken. In fact, battery-raised, commercially bred chicken is probably the worst meat of all. It ensures a product dosed with chemicals, hormones, and antibiotics. As if that weren't enough, it is now commonly recognized that there is a frightening incidence (four out of ten sold in the supermarket) of salmonella poisoning in much of today's chicken. Salmonella is strongly suspected in the dramatic increase in domestic food poisoning over the past few years—4 million cases of illness and 5,000 deaths in 1986. Some of you may have seen the "60 Minutes" documentary on the subject. If that didn't scare you off chicken, I don't know what will.

Fish would be the least dangerous of the animal proteins if not for today's contaminated seas, rivers, and lakes. Chemicals and additives are also routinely applied in fish farming practices. Fish does not represent a viable substitute either.

Your Best Alternatives

If you go on eating large quantities of animal protein on a daily basis, you will end up paying for it—maybe sooner, maybe later.

If you find it impossible to give it up completely, weigh your options. Choose those products that have the fewest additives and contaminants pumped into them. Look for sources of organic beef or chicken. Most American lamb grazes in areas free from chemical fertilizers and represents perhaps the least adulterated meat available on a commercial basis. As for fish, go for deep-sea varieties, which are farther from inshore pollution, such as red snapper, haddock, or mackerel. Choose small fish over big ones. Contaminants that cannot be assimilated get stored in the tissues of fish. Big fish eat smaller ones, thus absorbing more toxins. A tuna is likely to be far more toxic than a herring. Crustaceans (lobster, shrimp, mussels, scallops, crab, clams) should be treated with great caution. Most are harvested close to shore, some in highly contaminated environments. As scavengers, shellfish tend to feed on concentrations of contaminated waste and store what they cannot process.

So for you diehard meat eaters, when you eat animal protein, always accompany it with a big green salad and tomatoes, which will tend to neutralize the uric acid. Try not to eat animal protein on successive days; this will give your body a chance to regenerate itself.

2. REFINED SUGAR

The body needs sugar for energy, but the natural and rightful source of sugar is fruit and, to a lesser extent, certain vegetables. Sugar from these natural sources is rich in vitamins, minerals, and enzymes, which the body uses to assimilate and store the sugar.

What the body does not need is white refined sugar in any form. According to the USDA, the average American diet is almost 10 percent sugar—much of it hidden in foods and drinks not normally associated with sugar such as frozen foods, breads, cereals, mayonnaise, and salad dressings. In practice, this means (incredible as it may sound) that the average American consumes about 130 pounds of absolutely worthless and demonstrably dangerous sugar per year, or almost three pounds a week.

Refined sugar gives you a spurt of energy but is devoid of any nutritive value. It forms acids that cannot be utilized by the body and wreaks havoc in the nervous and endocrine systems. When eaten in combination with other foods, as it is when you have dessert after a meal, it also interferes with the digestive system. Sugar obstructs calcium metabolism, which is why it's so bad for your bones and your teeth. It is a direct cause of diabetes and of kidney, liver, and skin problems. Sugar has also been indicted as the chief culprit in hyperactive children and is linked to schizophrenia and dyslexia. It alters normal heart function. It gives you calories unaccompanied by any virtue. It is a food without a saving grace.

There are some authorities who hold the advertising industry to blame for the widespread overconsumption of sugar, but in fact, sugar does not need a publicist to make it attractive. It contains its own little devil within. Sugar is addictive. I mean this quite literally. Giving up or cutting down on sugar is even more difficult for my patients than giving up or cutting down on meat, dairy products and the other foods they ought to be doing without. It's ironic that the one food that has absolutely no beneficial properties whatsoever is the most difficult to give up. When people hooked on sugar try to quit cold turkey, they suffer withdrawal symptoms similar to those experienced by drug addicts (although less severe). Such people are literally sugar junkies. Unfortunately, most of us get addicted in early childhood. Many processed baby foods and commercial cereals contain sugar, and even the most diligent parents have trouble keeping sugar from their children.

Corn syrup and other sweeteners are not any better than sugar. They are the same—just sweet, dangerous calories. Meanwhile, the sugar substitutes—saccharin, aspartame (NutraSweet), and cyclamates—are no solution, despite advertising agency claims. They are chemicals, with no nutritive value. Yes, some have been approved by the FDA, but many substances that were once approved are now recognized as dangerous. Considerable controversy surrounds these sugar substitutes, and many tests incriminate them in a variety of lethal conditions. Giving up sugar and starting on sugar substitutes is a bit like kicking the heroin habit and becoming an alcoholic.

Isn't There Anything Sweet I Can Eat?

There is nothing sweet that you can eat with absolute impunity. Blackstrap molasses, the first stage of refined sugarcane, still contains most of its nutrients and in limited quantities is positively beneficial. (Raw sugarcane munched on by Caribbean children is a marvelous food and, amazingly, does not seem to cause cavities.) Raw, uncooked, untampered-with honey is also fine. Date sugar, 100 percent maple syrup, and other natural, unprocessed sugars all make acceptable sugar substitutes. But use them sparingly! Sweet dried fruits such as dates, figs, apricots, raisins, and currants are better for you and your kids than a Ding Dong or a Twinkie. But even these highly nutritious fruits are concentrated and should not be overindulged in.

3. COFFEE

Like refined sugar, coffee is absolutely devoid of nutritional value and is also addictive. As everyone knows, it's the caffeine that does it. The jolt from coffee goes right through your body. Caffeine is a drug, a nerve stimulant. It causes the heart to beat faster and increases the pulse rate and blood pressure. Respiration speeds up, kidneys are irritated, and the brain is stimulated, temporarily relieving fatigue or depression. But you pay dearly for this "hit," especially if you are an inveterate three-cup-or-more-a-day devotee. In the long term, caffeine strains the heart, prevents utilization of iron, causes vitamin deficiencies, and increases blood cholesterol. In addition, caffeine severely irritates the nervous system—it's like whipping a tired horse instead of giving it rest and a good meal. The trembling hands and tottering gait of many senior citizens is due in part to caffeine damaging their nervous systems. It's the end result of a lifetime of coffee nerves.

It's not just the caffeine that's the problem with coffee. It contains many other toxic substances that adversely affect the stomach, liver, heart, nervous system, and kidneys. Its powerful, volatile oils irritate the bowels. This is what brings about coffee's laxative effect in many people.

What About Coffee Substitutes?

Tea isn't really a substitute, since it also contains caffeine. Tea is just as bad as coffee, if not worse. It contains tannic acid, a powerful diuretic that sooner or later damages the delicate kidneys. Decaffeinated coffee isn't the answer either. Most of the caffeine may be gone, but enough remains to make it a toxic beverage that puts a strain on the kidneys. In addition, some decaffeinated coffee is treated with chemicals known to be carcinogens.

Kicking the Coffee Habit

Because coffee is addictive, it will be difficult to give up. But it can be done. What is it you like about coffee? The pick-me-up? Your body does not need false stimulants and will eventually rebel against them. The good news is that once you modify your diet, you won't need that pick-me-up. Start the day with dry skin brushing and a fresh-fruit breakfast, and see how unnecessary that morning cup of coffee becomes.

Is it the taste you love? The heady aroma? Try Caffix, Yanoh, or Pero, all coffee substitutes derived from cereal. While not exactly good for you, they're better than coffee and at least approximate the smell and taste. Many of my patients find that a cup of hot water with a couple of teaspoons of blackstrap molasses and a squeeze of lemon makes a good coffee substitute. But maybe it's the warm, cozy feeling of drinking a cup of coffee you love. Try a nice cup of herbal tea instead. There are many different types available in health food stores, herb shops—even supermarkets. They are easy to make and tasty. Adding a little honey and lemon can enhance their flavor still further.

If you simply can't break the habit, try a thick wedge of lemon squeezed into black coffee. It will tend to neutralize the effects of caffeine and ease the transition to total abstinence. Try to cut back on the amount you drink until you can break the habit completely.

4. FATS AND OILS

All oils should be used sparingly. Most Americans grossly over-consume oils, and the wrong oils at that. Cold-pressed crude virgin oils from vegetable sources provide essential unsaturated fats (vitamin F) that help keep arteries resilient. The best oils are cold-pressed sesame, olive, and avocado. Other acceptable oils are sunflower, safflower, corn, and soy.

Hydrogenated fats or shortenings, though vegetable-based, are heated and hardened in order to lengthen their shelf life. In the process they are turned into substances the digestive system does not readily assimilate. In this class are oleomargarine, commercial mayonnaise, and hydrogenated salted or sweetened peanut butter. (Fresh-ground peanut butter from the health food store is preferable, but all peanut butter is acid-forming and hard to digest. I mix peanut butter in equal parts with sesame tahini, which tastes marvelous and obviates most of the problems associated with peanut butter. Try other nut butters instead of peanut butter. Almond butter is the best.)

Fortunately, people no longer rely heavily upon animal fats (lard, bacon drippings, etc.) in cooking. Even the hydrogenated fats are better than these animal products. On the other hand, pure sweet butter (raw is the ideal and can sometimes be found in health food stores) is perfectly acceptable when used with discretion. For cooking use stick butter; for eating use sweet whipped butter. The whipping process breaks down the butter's fat globules, allowing the liver to assimilate it more easily.

Heated fats tend to adhere to the walls of the arteries. Other foods then build up on this fatty coating (cholesterol is the best known, but calcium from milk and cheese do also). Narrowing and hardening of the arteries are the eventual result. So all fried foods should be eaten very sparingly and deep-fried foods should be eaten more sparingly still. (This means french fries!) Reused frying oils go rancid in the reheating process and become carcinogenic. Since even those restaurants that use quality oils reuse those oils, it is a good practice to avoid all restaurant fried food.

It's impossible to overestimate the amount of damage done to American health by overconsumption of fats. On the plus side, the damage done by fats can be overcome by conscientiously increasing the amount of green leafy vegetables you eat. So if you find it nearly impossible to give up favorite fried foods, treat yourself to massive salad doses on the side and you won't be doing yourself much harm. This applies especially to the kids. Make a rule: No fried junk without a salad before, with, or after.

5. MILK AND MILK PRODUCTS

Milk is a source of calcium, minerals, and vitamins. But to contend that it is *the* source, the best source, or even a good source of these nutrients is a gross misrepresentation of the facts, an act of unpardonable irresponsibility by the dairy industry.

If children are breast-fed to the age of two or three, they will have no further need of milk. If children are weaned earlier, they will certainly have to get their calcium from somewhere, but that somewhere ought not to be cow's milk—especially not tasteless, pasteurized, homogenized cow's milk. Pasteurized milk is dead milk. It is devoid of many enzymes and antibodies that children need.

Cow's milk is hard to digest, and it gets harder the older you get. The reason is that we lose the enzymes to digest it. Many adults develop a positive, even virulent intolerance to milk products. Because of the missing enzyme (lactose), milk is not digested. It ferments within the system and becomes a toxic substance, leading to allergies, gas, skin problems, mucus formation, and respiratory and digestive disorders. It also acts as a laxative or cathartic and provokes diarrhea. As if that weren't enough, milk is a major contributor to arthritis and hardening of the arteries. One of the first things I advise my arthritic patients is to avoid all milk and milk products. It is very rare that they do not quickly show improvement.

Certified whole raw milk is much less harmful than pasteurized milk. Goat's milk is better still. It's the nearest thing to mother's milk furnished by nature. Like all milk products, it is to be used sparingly. I put patients with serious digestive problems on goat's milk temporarily, until the body revitalizes enough to allow them to handle other foods.

Gee Whiz Doc, What About Cheese, Yogurt, and Sour Cream?

Good yogurt in moderation isn't bad. The process of turning milk into cheese makes cheese more digestible. In limited amounts it supplies protein, and this is particularly important to certain people who may have difficulty assimilating protein from vegetable sources. Sour cream? I wouldn't have borscht without it. But I mix it in equal parts with yogurt. The secret is caution. Eat sparingly. Learn your own tolerances. Don't be a fanatic about it.

Where Will I Get Calcium?

You can get all the calcium you need without any digestive or allergic problems from broccoli, corn, oatmeal, sesame seeds, most raw nuts (especially almonds), millet, molasses, dates, kelp, dulse, and all green leafy vegetables. In fact, if you are eating at all reasonably, you would have to go well out of your way to find foods that would *not* supply you with all the calcium you need.

6. SALT

Salt is an inorganic substance that irritates your delicate nervous system and mucous membranes. To the best of my knowledge, salt has no nutrient effect whatsoever (except to replace some mineral salts lost through excessive perspiration in very hot weather). When salt is taken into the body, the body's response is to get rid of it as soon as possible. It surrounds the salt with liquid and expels it through the kidneys. This is why you feel so thirsty after eating salty food. The body has excreted large quantities of fluid in order to get rid of the salt. Too much salt often results in hypertension and may lead to a severe kidney affliction called *nephritis*. Everybody's intake of salt should be drastically reduced or eliminated altogether. That delicious salty taste can be satisfactorily reproduced with kelp and dulse mixed with a little sea salt (to supply needed iodine). Check your health food store for vegetable-based seasonings that can be used as salt substitutes.

7. REFINED GRAINS

Your daily bread today resembles a finished laboratory product more than a bakery product and is, according to some prominent nutritionists, not the staff of life but of death.

Today's white bread—presliced, bleached, and stuffed with chemicals—is an abomination, with ingredients that read more like a chemical prescription and would be more at home in a pharmacy or laboratory than on a grocery or supermarket shelf. What a joy to unwrap that appealing crisp wrapper and to sink your teeth into all that acetic acid, lactic acid, potassium tartrate, ascorbic acid (synthetic vitamin C), monocalcium sulfate, sodium diacetate, potassium bromate, sodium propionate, sodium phosphate, ammonium sulfate, potassium sulfate, chlorine dioxide, sulfur dioxide, glycerol monostearate, and calcium propionate! Yes, the white bread you and your family eat year in and year out is responsible, according to researchers, for many human ailments.

At one time millers ground wheat between large stones turned by windmill sails. They would then send the ground flour to the baker, who lovingly kneaded the dough before placing it in his oven, from which it would emerge as a crisp, delicious feast fit for a king.

The miller and his windmill have long since been replaced by technicians and giant machines in "flour mills" bearing little relation to the stone mills of old. The modern mill is where most of the "chemicalization" of flour takes place. A laboratory scientist now cooks up new preservatives, softeners, emulsifiers, and stabilizers that end up in our daily bread.

Modern, mass-produced bread is a far cry from the delicious-smelling, tasty, crusty whole-grain or rye breads still baked in some homes and small "natural" bakeries from such simple ingredients as oats, whole wheat, whole rye, millet, soy flour, yeast, and water.

Tampering with Bread

Tampering started many years ago, when the manufacturers, the new "bakers," found that the calcium in flour disintegrated if it was stored too long. The texture of bread was adversely affected. So they replaced this calcium with calcium carbonate (chalk), the first of a never-ending line of additives: ascorbic acid, potassium bromate, ammonium sulfate, potassium sulfate, chlorine dioxide, benzoyl peroxide, and, in some flours, chlorine and sulfur dioxide. The primary purpose of these chemicals was to bleach the flour snow white and to give the finished loaf that "light, fluffy" texture. Then the manufacturers pumped in various acids to preserve the breads for longer shelf life: acetic acid (vinegar), sodium phosphate, lactic acid, potassium tartrates, and sodium diacetate. Now the manufacturers had a product that was white and fluffy and had eye appeal and a longer shelf life. There was only one problem: it had no nutritional value. All the good stuff disappeared with the wheat germ and bran that had been thrown out to produce that white, fluffy, advertisable loaf.

The germ contains many valuable nutrients, including most of the B group and vitamin E. Because the most nutritious elements were being destroyed or discarded, the federal government insisted by law that some of the more important vitamins and minerals, such as B_1 and iron, be replaced. Hence "fortified bread." Unfortunately, this does not include other valuable nutrients that are normally present in all whole-grain flour. Significantly, when a baker bakes whole-grain bread, he is not required by law to add anything, so most of the original vitamins and minerals are naturally present. Whole-grain bread also contains bran, and latest medical research into bowel complaints (including diverticular disease of the bowel) suggests that the large increase of these ailments may be due to a widespread decline of roughage in the national diet.

Why Gluten Is Harmful

Gluten is the protein part of the wheat. It is a tough, sticky, nitrogenous substance. Most grains, especially wheat, oatmeal, and barley, are high in gluten. When you eat gluten it gradually forms mucus, which coats the villi—those tiny fingers that stick out from the wall of the small intestine and absorb nutrients from the primarily liquid digested food. But when the villi are heavily coated with mucus they cannot absorb the nutrients, and so they do not get

through to the body. Over a period of time gluten builds up like a
plastic film in your small intestine and seriously interferes with food
assimilation. It also gradually erodes the myelin sheath (the outer
coating or skin of every nerve in the body) and eventually "short-
circuits" your nerves.

Some of the products with the highest gluten content are among
America's favorite (and also most dangerous) foods. Pizza, pretzels,
bagels, bialys, and pitas are almost nothing but gluten. Eaten on a
regular basis, these foods will clog up the digestive system and set
you up for future disease. You may eat large quantities of wheat
for decades with no problem, but the chances are if you do not cut
down, eventually it will catch up with you in the form of digestive
and/or nervous disorders.

In recent years the prevalence of wheat and grain allergies has
been recognized. Many mysterious skin, respiratory, and digestive
allergies have been traced to wheat and other gluten-rich grains. It
went undetected for so long because most of us eat wheat and wheat
products so often that nobody thought to look into it as the possible
cause.

What About Switching to Whole Wheat or Rye?

Whole wheat bread is certainly rich in nutrients and rich in taste,
but as far as the gluten is concerned, it is no better than white bread.
The popular Jewish rye has more wheat in it than is good for you,
as does pumpernickel. Both should be eaten sparingly. Sourdough
rye with minimal wheat content is much better, as are sprouted rye,
corn bread, soy bread, and mixed-grain bread.

The message is clear. Cut way back on gluten-rich foods,
difficult as that may be. In practice, I find that most people have a
certain tolerance for wheat. Some of my patients tell me they can
handle a sandwich and a half and feel no ill effects, but if they have
two sandwiches, the effect is dramatic. The stomach bloats or their
eyes swell, sneezing or coughing spells may occur, or it hits their
sinuses; others come down with skin rashes or bad digestion. If you
have trouble digesting your morning toast or pancakes, it means
your body is protesting against the gluten onslaught.

8. DRINKING WATER

There are nearly as many types of water as there are uses for it. Most tap water comes from streams, rivers, and reservoirs. This surface water often contains pollutants and agricultural wastes, such as fertilizer and insecticide residue, that are carried by rainwater runoff into nearby waterways. Unfortunately, in the past few decades our water supplies have been endangered by hundreds of new chemicals and pollutants every year. In addition, water-treatment facilities have not kept technological pace with the techniques necessary to neutralize or remove increasing contamination.

A few years ago the National Research Council reported that so little is known about so many pollutants that safe levels for them are almost impossible to set. Modern laboratories are now equipped to identify specific chemicals in terms of billionths of parts of water being tested. In certain cases scientists can measure in the *trillionths*. These figures are almost inconceivable for a layperson. But in case you think that such small amounts are insignificant, keep in mind that one can become quite ill from a single microscopic particle of some contaminant.

"I Picked Up a Bug Somewhere."

What is the effect of consuming contaminants over long periods of time? We know that acute, immediate illness usually comes from a virus or a poison, but chronic, long-term problems that develop over many years are diagnosed less readily. The scientific community is genuinely concerned that prolonged exposure to certain elements, even at low levels, may be a factor in the increasing incidence of cancer and heart disease. Even "intestinal flu"—headaches, fever, nausea, and diarrhea—may be picked up in your drinking water. And intestinal flu or gastroenteritis may be the least of many ailments transmitted by water.

Is water a source of cancer? Is water a source of birth defects? Is water a source of genetic mutations? Is water innocent on all these counts? No one is certain. Most Americans believe that our drinking water is pure. There are so many exceptions, however, that in 1974 the U.S. Congress had to enact special legislation to ensure that our water was reasonably safe.

We do know there are two substances in your drinking water that pose an immediate threat to your health whenever the standards that have been set for them are exceeded:

> • *Bacteria*. Coliform bacteria from human and animal waste may sometimes be found in drinking water. Waterborne diseases such as typhoid, cholera, infectious hepatitis, and dysentery have been traced to drinking water contaminated by bacteria. Should you ever receive notice that the bacteria level in your water exceeds the minimum standard, follow directions given in the notice.
> • *Nitrates*. These substances in drinking water above the national standard pose an immediate threat to children under three months of age. In some infants, excessive levels of nitrates react with hemoglobin in the blood to produce an anemic condition commonly known as blue baby. If you receive notice that your drinking water contains an excessive amount of nitrate, do not give this water to an infant under three months of age and do not use it to prepare baby formulas. Never boil water, as boiling increases the nitrate concentration. Simply read the notice you receive and follow the instructions carefully.

To make New York City water sparkle, I have heard that Calgon, a dishwasher detergent, is added in minute doses. But this is the least of the problems. Between the time the rains fall from the heavens and the time you drink them from a glass, as many as sixty other chemicals may be added. Among them: chlorine (to kill bacteria), fluorine (to prevent tooth decay), lime (to neutralize acidic water and retard corrosion in pipes), copper sulfate (to kill algae), aluminum sulfate (to coagulate and settle out particles), sodium bisulfate or sulfur dioxide (to neutralize an overdose of chlorine).

Water naturally contains many minerals and chemicals. Some can be injurious to health even as they occur in nature. But in 1980 the government's Council on Environmental Quality reported specifically on man-tampered water, citing an increased risk of urinary tract and gastrointestinal cancer from chlorinated water. Major water supplies to avoid are those of New Orleans, Atlantic City, and Miami. My suggestion to you, if you are interested in improving your health, is to drink distilled water (*not* spring water).

Distilled Water vs. Spring Water

As mentioned earlier, distilled water is water that has been boiled and converted to steam, and then recondensed. In this process, everything that is not pure hydrogen and oxygen is removed. The result is pure water. In the human body, this acts as a solvent to help clean out the arteries, lungs, liver, and kidneys.

Spring water comes from a well, a spring, or a river, and it's full of hard, inorganic minerals that accumulate in the body. Rain-water, in percolating down through the soil into a spring or well, picks up minerals along the way that are held in suspension in the water. Your body cannot break these substances down and use them in this inorganic form. When a fruit or vegetable picks up these minerals, it digests them, and that is how they become organic. When you eat the fruit or the vegetable, you're getting organic, plant-digested minerals, which your body can easily digest and assimilate. If you have any health problems, drink distilled water exclusively. This alone will make a big difference in your health. Indeed, all liquid that enters your body, whether it's tea or soup, should be made with distilled water. (For bathing or washing, ordinary water is fine.)

9. VINEGAR

Vinegar is a fermented liquid that should not be classed as a food. It actually interferes with and slows down digestion. It is also a powerful irritant. Along with alcohol, it is described as a protoplasmic poison that destroys red blood cells and the functioning power of the brain. Vinegar is much easier to give up than many other avoidable foods. Fresh lemon or lime juice easily replaces it.

10. GARLIC AND ONION

Both garlic and onion have valuable antiseptic properties. But raw, they are irritants. When you cut a raw onion, your eyes tear because the delicate mucous membranes have been irritated by the powerful mustardlike gas released by the onion. Obviously the mucous membranes within the body cannot help but react in similar fashion. The irritant properties disappear in cooking, while some of the antiseptic properties are retained. Raw garlic and onions can be soaked in lemon juice or overnight in water to get rid of the irritants. The moral: Go easy on untreated raw garlic and raw onions. Your body and all your friends will be grateful.

11. GRANOLA

Granola is made up of various mixtures of grains and shares their virtues and their vices. Though high in B vitamins and minerals, it is also high in gluten; it is acid-forming and commercial brands are usually sweetened with low-grade honey.

I do find that granola makes a useful transition food. Patients who cannot face giving up all their gluten habits in one fell swoop can wean themselves relatively painlessly and harmlessly with granola. Look for a mix high in raw millet, buckwheat groats, and corn, and low in wheat and rice. A good idea is to make your own. The ingredients are readily available in health food stores. Sweeten and moisten granola with apple juice or soy milk, never with cow's milk.

12. CEREAL

Apart from their high gluten content, most commercial cereals have been treated with preservatives and antiworm chemicals at some stage in their manufacture. Grains may also be stored for years before reaching the table, and there is no law against it. The longer grains are stored, the more nutrients they lose. Millet, whole brown rice, cornmeal, buckwheat groats, and cream of rye are the best cereals.

13. BREWER'S YEAST

Although brewer's yeast is rich in B vitamins and temporarily stimulating, it is vastly overrated. It contains a specific uric-acid-like substance that makes it more acid-forming than almost any other available vegetable-derived food. Its B vitamins may be obtained from rice bran, rice polish, or oat bran.

14. EGGPLANT

Considerable controversy surrounds the eggplant. Some nutritionists and vegetarians swear by it. There is, however, no doubt that eggplant contains a substance that constricts the heart muscle and arteries around the heart in many people. As vegetables go, it is also surprisingly low in nutritional value, though it has traces of many vitamins and minerals. To my mind the minuses outweigh the pluses. Eat it sparingly or, if you're allergic, not at all.

15. ALCOHOL

The ill effects of alcohol, especially when taken in excess, are so well known that they hardly bear repetition here. Apart from the intrinsic dangers associated with alcohol, the problem today is compounded by massive additions of chemicals, especially to wine and beer. Over a million people have allergies traced to these additives, but there is no way for them to know specifically what they are reacting to, since distillers, brewers, and vintners are not obliged to list ingredients on their products.

16. HOSPITAL FOOD

According to C. E. Butterworth, M.D., the chairman of the Council on Foods and Nutrition of the American Medical Association, writing in *Nutrition Today*, "One of the largest pockets of unrecognized malnutrition in America and Canada, too, exists not in rural slums or urban ghettos, but in the private rooms and wards of big city hospitals."

This is no joke. There is probably no place in the world with lower nutritional standards and worse cooks than hospitals. Hospital food is idiotically planned, horribly overcooked, and presents a major factor in preventing or impeding recovery. People who manage to get well after several weeks or more on a hospital diet provide another testament to the wonderful resilience of the human body.

If you find yourself in the hospital for more than a couple of days, you should take the matter of hospital food seriously. Your recovery, and even your life, may depend upon it. The first line of defense is of course not to go through the standard menu. Most hospitals will be happy to serve you baked potatoes for lunch and dinner and even breakfast. A baked potato is one of the most nutritious foods you can find anywhere. The hospital will also give you fresh fruit, if you ask for it, and a salad, though this is likely to contain the least nutritious of all salad greens—iceberg lettuce.

Your second line of defense is friends and family. They can bring salads, millet, fruit, whatever. So don't despair. Even if you must go to the hospital, you are not obliged to eat the food. Remember, you are in the hospital because your body has been through a shock or trauma, possibly life-threatening. Your body requires low-stress, high-nutrition food so that all its energy can be devoted to healing rather than digesting.

CHAPTER 10

Staying Healthy in a Poisoned World

New health magazines sprout everywhere, health food stores and health cooperatives do land-office business—even the medical profession is becoming aware of the nutrition disease connection. But the fact is, we live in a poisoned world. Most of our disease is the result of stress. Deliberately or accidentally, our bodies are going through hard times. The principles and practices of natural healing are hard to apply in our "civilized" society. I believe the American public should know exactly how the dice are loaded against natural healing. In this chapter I will outline the major political and social conditions that conspire against your health and mine.

Let's imagine the life of an infant born to Mr. and Mrs. Average American and trace the numerous obstacles to be overcome:

1. Breast feeding is back in fashion. But a very large percentage of new mothers cannot afford to leave the work force to stay home and breast-feed, and others can't be bothered. So there's a good chance our average baby will be fed from the bottle, even though everyone knows better. There is only one proper food for the human baby, and that is milk from its mother's breast. As we know, breast milk is far superior to bottled milk. Through it a healthy mother passes her immunity on to her child. Cow's milk, formulas based upon cow's milk, and even soy-based formulas do not and cannot

replace mother's milk. Cow's milk is overladen with protein and deficient in absorbable calcium. Studies have shown that children raised on cow's milk tend to be taller but also that there is a correlation between increased height and decreased health and longevity. Soy-based formulas contain milk sugar and/or chemical additives that your baby was not designed to drink. The baby was designed to drink breast milk. Moreover, the act of breast feeding is essential for creating the mother/child bond that will ultimately result in happy family relationships. The child cannot develop a relationship with the bottle.

For those infants who are breast-fed, there are still problems. Breast milk from an unhealthy mother is as bad as, if not worse than, cow's milk or formula. Mothers who are on drugs, mothers who are on medication, mothers who smoke or drink, and mothers who are junk food junkies are doing their babies no favor by breast feeding.

NOTE: Certified raw milk, that is to say, milk that has not had all its nutrients cooked out of it in the pasteurization process, makes an acceptable substitute for mother's milk on a temporary basis or in an emergency (physical debility or unavoidable social circumstances). Those living in rural areas with access to certified raw milk can use it, assured they will not be doing their baby damage.

2. Since the majority of babies are born in cities and suburbs, our average baby will live in an atmosphere polluted by diesel and gasoline fumes, heavy sulfur concentrations, and industrial chemicals and poisons too numerous for the EPA to keep track of. There is no such thing as an unpolluted American city. The situation in rural areas is better, but not by much. Scarcely a week goes by without some new study showing that some poison or carcinogen is leaching its way into what appears to be lovely countryside or even pristine wilderness.

3. The water the baby drinks will most likely be strongly chemicalized. All city drinking supplies have chemicals added to make them "safe" to drink—which is not to say it makes them fit to drink! Country dwellers are scarcely better off. According to a recent EPA study, 63% of rural residents may drink water contaminated with pesticides. Universally contaminated water supplies represent one of the more horrible surprises of the past decade (see page 224). Small wonder that bottled water is one of America's

major growth industries, but who wants to bet that this water from mountain springs is free from pollutants raining down over every square inch of the earth's surface? Not me.

4. The baby will most likely be fed baby food, which is not food in any meaningful sense of the word. It's highly processed, and any nutritional value has disappeared in the processing. It cannot be otherwise. And many brands contain sugar. What's more, to pay for all the advertising, those little bottles don't cost much less than the equivalent amount of caviar. (Eat well yourself and feed your baby what you eat.)

5. As soon as the baby has reached toddler stage, he or she takes his or her place at the table with Mom and Dad. Junior is pumped full of the usual combination of too much animal protein, too much fat, too much sugar, too much salt, and not enough of anything that is actually nourishing. The worst part of all of this is that Junior likes it. His or her senses are perverted from the very beginning. The habit is as difficult to break as narcotics. In my opinion, McDonald's should be as illegal as cocaine. What's more, Junior grows up thinking that all of this is normal: coffee, cigarettes, tea, alcohol, soda pop, junk food . . . and of course, illness everywhere.

6. When the child reaches school age, the nutritional onslaught continues. Most school lunches are influenced by federal government and American Dietetic Association standards. While it is true that children do not show much culinary discrimination, school food still represents an insult to both their stomachs and their intelligence, and all kids know it. Local papers commonly publish school menus. Follow them for a week or two yourself and see what the kids are getting—an overload of animal protein, and low-grade protein at that. They are not getting steaks, fresh fish, or roast chicken; they are getting grilled hot dogs, pepperoni pizzas, chicken patties, and hamburgers. Surely you remember what a school hamburger tasted like.*

---

*In order to balance the national budget in the early 1980s, the Reagan administration, with David Stockman leading the fight, proposed considering ketchup a vegetable in the children's school lunch program. This was so ludicrous it caused an immediate outcry.

At school Junior will also be subjected to significant amounts of stress, both subtle and damaging. "Peer pressure" is one label applied to it, but it's more than that. It's the whole educational system itself, which drums useless rubbish into kids' heads, forcing them to learn (by rote) information devoid of educational significance, and obliges them to spend long hours doing homework in the process. In a sane society learning is a pleasure; in ours it is a chore. It is a wonder that any children grow up even reasonably healthy or happy, and in fact, not many do.

7. Time not spent in homework or at school is likely to be spent in front of the tube. This applies particularly to latchkey children and children from single-parent families. The poor children are subjected to a barrage of marketing and public relations campaigns. Effectively, they are being brainwashed into thinking that everything bad for them is good for them. It's as simple as that. What is at stake are the profit margins of giant corporations whose financial health is more important than the physical or mental health of our children.

The fact of the matter is, there isn't much out there in the modern world that *isn't* opposed to the principles of natural healing. It's almost a built-in antagonism. The aims and goals of big business and natural healing are intrinsically in conflict. It seems to me that an almost unimaginable change of heart or conscience would be required before business interests and health interests work toward the same goals. I don't say it's impossible, but even with the new focus on health and fitness, it's a long way from happening. Here are just a few of the vested interests involved (some obvious and some not so obvious):

- The chemical industry: manufacturers of fertilizers, insecticides, and pesticides
- Distilleries, vintners, and brewers
- The livestock industry
- The baking industry
- The tobacco industry
- The cosmetic industry
- The condiment, spice, and salt manufacturers
- The supermarket chains

- The sugar refiners
- The tea, coffee, and cocoa industry
- The multinational pharmaceutical corporations
- The medical profession

When you see what is at stake and who is involved, you don't have to be a genius or a prophet to understand the problem. How can governments seriously promote natural healing or try to further the natural health movement on a nationwide or worldwide scale? Every government in the world is sustained by financial and commercial interests and economic considerations hostile to the fundamental goals of natural healing. It is not that big business or Big Brother is deliberately trying to make people sick; it's just that no one, myself included, can think of a way of promoting real health and well-being on a nationwide scale without undermining or even destroying major industries. But the fact remains that the government is often put into a position of helping these industries at our expense. The great "All-American Breakfast" is one obvious example of this.

Inventing the Importance of the All-American Breakfast

You probably think a hearty breakfast is essential to good health. Americans have thought that for three generations. But the truth is that the All-American Breakfast is an invention cooked up during the Great Depression. People were starving, but at the same time there was a glut of grain, and farmers couldn't unload their harvest. Roosevelt called in his famous "brain trust"—the brilliant Harry Hopkins, Felix Frankfurter, and Thomas Corcoran ("Tommy the Cork")—along with Bernard Bernays, the father of public relations. They mulled over the problem for weeks and then found the answer: the All-American Breakfast. They called all the newspapers, publishers, and magazines, and invited the editors to Washington. I was around at the time, and I remember it well. Not long after that, articles began appearing trumpeting the virtues of a hearty breakfast. The word was out that breakfast was the most important meal of the day, and the All-American Breakfast was born.

Now people ate breakfast before that, of course. And some people ate substantial breakfasts. But this insistence upon breakfast as the most important meal of the day—that was new, and it was and is pure hype. No one has ever demonstrated the necessity or even the advisability of a big breakfast. But so brilliant was the campaign that it's only in the last few years that nutritionists have begun to question its conclusions, with near-unanimous results. We don't need a big breakfast. In fact, we don't need any breakfast. In my view one of the great best-kept secrets of health is to start the day with the lightest possible breakfast, and then only fruit. But better still is to avoid breakfast altogether.

Why? It's simple and logical. When you wake up in the morning you tend to have foul breath and a coated tongue. There is a good reason for this. Once your body has broken down and assimilated dinner and whatever snacks you may have had before going to bed, its energy is devoted to detoxifying and healing. That's the reason for the foul breath. This is waste eliminated by the lungs landing up on your tongue. When you eat your famous All-American Breakfast, you put a halt to the detoxifying/healing process, and for no reason. You don't need the energy; you've stored all the energy from last night's dinner. And in fact, if you have a really heavy bacon-and-eggs breakfast, you end up with less available energy than when you started because the body has to work so hard just to digest it. On the other hand, if you have no breakfast, the cleansing/detoxifying process continues unabated. Fruit will slow the process down somewhat but will also give you instant energy.

Yes, yes, I hear the protests and see the waving hands. What about all the studies that show that children who do not have a substantial breakfast do poorly in school? Well, I wonder who funded those studies. The *British Journal of Nutrition* came to an exactly opposite conclusion. According to this prestigious publication, there was absolutely no difference between the performance of children who ate big breakfasts and those who didn't. We should also keep in mind that in this country it's possible that kids who do not have a substantial breakfast have miserable lunches and dinners as well. It may simply be a question of general malnutrition. The point I want to make here is that the All-American Breakfast is a con job: a political and marketing invention, not only unnecessary but actually detrimental to your health.

The government-recommended hearty breakfast is, like most governmental nutritional guidelines, misconceived. In this case and in many others, these guidelines are positively detrimental to the nation's health and beneficial only to the nation's supermarkets.

The Standard American Diet (SAD)

Here is what your government tells you to eat (these are called "conventional" foods):

1. The milk and dairy group, consisting of two servings daily of one cup of milk, eight ounces of yogurt, one and a half ounces of natural cheese, or two ounces of processed cheese. (Three servings for teens and for women who are pregnant or breastfeeding; four servings for teens who are pregnant or breastfeeding.)

2. Meat, poultry, fish, and alternatives (eggs, dry beans and peas, nuts, and seeds), consisting of two to three servings daily of five to seven ounces of lean meat, fish, or poultry. Count one egg, one half cup cooked dry beans, or two tablespoons of peanut butter as one ounce of lean meat.

3. The bread, cereal, and other grain products group, consisting of six to eleven daily servings (including several servings a day of whole-grain products) of one slice of bread; one-half hamburger bun or English muffin; a small roll, biscuit, or muffin; three to four small or two large crackers; one-half cup cooked cereal, rice, or pasta; or one ounce of ready-to-eat breakfast cereal.

4. The fruits group, consisting of two to four daily servings of a piece of whole fruit, such as an apple, banana, or orange; a grapefruit half; a melon wedge; three quarters of a cup of juice; one-half cup berries; or one-half cup cooked or canned fruit; or one-quarter cup dried fruit.

5. The vegetables group, consisting of three to five servings of one-half cup of cooked or chopped raw vegetables or one cup of leafy raw vegetables, such as lettuce or spinach. (All vegetable types included regularly, dark-green leafy vegetables and dry beans and peas several times a week.)

6. Avoid too many fats and sweets. If you drink alcoholic beverages, do so in moderation.

The government may consider these dietary guidelines. It is their recommendation for a Standard American Diet. I call it S.A.D. If you study it closely, you will find it grossly overemphasizes proteins, grains, and dairy products, and sells short fresh fruits, vegetables, and alternative protein sources. It promotes overcooked, acid-forming, toxic foods without even a clue to the crucial importance of food combining. Over a period of time SAD can only lead to degenerative, chronic disease, general malaise, universal obesity, and richer doctors.

That was the bad news. Here's the worse news. The one food group not included in SAD is junk. In fact, junk food is the mainstay of the diet for many Americans, especially the young. Certainly most Americans include a large amount of junk food in their diets. Soda, candy, pastries, jams, jellies, cookies, potato chips, corn chips, snack foods, diet foods, and diet pop make up 50 percent of the diet of most Americans. Per capita consumption of soft drinks rose from 9.6 ounces a day in 1975 to 16 ounces in 1985. Forty percent of the nation's one-to-two-year-olds drink an average of 9 ounces of soft drinks a day. And the fastest growing breakfast item in America is soda, up 80 percent since 1983.

It was only in 1981 that researchers began looking for connections between cancer and nutrition. The latest figures from the Centers for Disease Control estimate that 35 percent of all cancers are nutrition-related. My own estimate would be at least 50 percent or more, and I would have made that estimate back in 1955, but nobody was listening then. To follow SAD is to court disaster. To follow the actual all-American diet is to ensure catastrophe.

Supermarket or Chemical Market?

Just stand at the checkout counter of your local supermarket and look at the junk in the carts. Walk down an aisle, any aisle, and pick up a selection of jars, cans, and bottles. Read the labels and count the chemicals—the ones you know and the ones you don't. It is an established fact that *none* of these chemicals promote good health, and many, in fact, are damaging to your health. New studies usually incriminate, and seldom exonerate, whatever chemical or additive may be under consideration. It would be naïve to blame the supermarkets directly. The supermarket is interested in making money, not in promoting good health.

If people insisted upon chemical-free, organically grown produce, the supermarkets would stock it very swiftly. The recent appearance of salad bars in supermarkets—and now of sulfite-free salad bars—proves how sensitive the supermarkets can be to public demand. It would be equally naïve to expect better behavior from the food industry and the chemical industry, which are responsible for inventing these products with interminable shelf lives and infinitesimal nutritional value. They are also out to make money. The answer is not to eat their rubbish and to teach our children not to eat it either. But let's take a look at the additives, chemicals, and dyes without which there would be no processed food industry at all.

Two Thousand "Necessary" Additives

American food processors pump an estimated 2,400 food additives into their products. There are over 2,000 listed food flavorings. These additives fall into three categories:

1. Additives essential to a product's existence. Low-calorie drinks would be impossible without chemical sweeteners. Aerosol whipped toppings require chemical propellants. Some food products would actually be dangerous without additives. (How dangerous they are with additives is a matter under dispute.)

2. Additives essential to a product's marketability. When you cook at home, do you add preservatives? Of course not. But preservatives are vital to the food manufacturer, who needs some way to keep his product from going bad long enough to produce it, get it to the supermarket, and store it until you are silly enough to buy it. Without added preservatives the whole process becomes impossible. And in fact, it's to the manufacturer's best interest to try to make his products keep forever. That way he never has to absorb the cost of replacing a product that has not been sold within its shelf life.

3. Additives that make the product more appealing to the eye. If processed food looked the way it tastes, who would dream of buying it? Hence the food dyes. Among the dyes permitted by the FDA, six are known carcinogens.

Mystery Meat

Closely related to the problem of additives in processed food is the universal incidence of additives in fresh food. The problem of pesticides and chemical fertilizers has been fairly well publicized, even though it has not yet been seriously addressed. The problem of livestock systematically stimulated by hormones and laced with antibiotics and known toxic drugs has only recently come to the attention of the general public. At stake is the 2-billion-dollar-a-year animal drug industry and the 70-billion-dollar-a-year livestock industry. It is not surprising, then, that action has not yet been taken. Meanwhile, the public is being exposed en masse to meats that not only contain dangerous substances but are dangerous in themselves. As noted earlier, nearly four out of ten chickens sold to consumers contain salmonella microorganisms, the agents responsible for a serious flulike fever. The routine use of antibiotics in animals results in proven human resistance to these drugs. In simple terms, this means that if you get an infection that requires antibiotics to cure it, you may not respond because you've built up an immunity through eating too much antibiotic-doctored meat. The widespread use of growth hormones has resulted in children reaching puberty at nine or ten years old.

So, when I strongly advise you to cut down drastically on all animal proteins, it is not just because alternative protein sources provide protein in less toxic and more assimilable forms. It is also because the animal protein we commonly get contains all manner of quite horrifying contaminants and additives. Moreover, as studies now show, we Americans simply eat too much protein in the first place, and it is making us sick. The myth that we need a high-protein diet is older than the myth of the Great American Breakfast, but equally without substance. A recent study from the National Academy of Sciences contends that excess protein may well be a factor in cancers of the breast, colon, rectum, pancreas, and kidney.

Food Irradiation

Recognizing the dangers of additives and preservatives and, what's more important, the marketing power of an alerted public, the food industry has now joined forces with the nuclear industry on a new gimmick that's even more ominous: food irradiation. Irradiation preserves food without chemical additives by exposing it to radiation derived from nuclear waste. They're saving us from the dangers of chemical additives by substituting low-level radioactivity. And it's not just that exposure to radiation is inherently dangerous. Irradiation, while it does kill the microbes and insects that infect food from the outside, also alters and destroys the ripening enzymes within the food, upsetting and deranging its molecular structure. DNA, which is the vital life force in food, becomes unbalanced, along with the enzymes or living protein. An irradiated banana, for example, looks like any other banana, but in fact it is sterile, since it has been changed molecularly.

What is at stake is the safety of your food and mine. Extensive tests have been run showing that rats fed irradiated food in laboratory tests died. Children in India fed irradiated wheat developed blood abnormalities. Mice fed irradiated chicken developed genital cancers. Incredibly, the FDA has ignored these studies and pronounced food irradiation safe.

As if the danger from the process were not terrifying enough, there is an added threat in food irradiation. In order to implement it on the commercial scale envisioned by both government and industry, nuclear processing plants (proven safe, of course—remember Chernobyl and Three Mile Island!) will have to be set up near many major urban sites. Meanwhile, in extracting the radioactive cesium 137 required for food irradiation, huge new stockpiles of weapons-grade plutonium will be created. This, according to food irradiation opponents (advocates are called experts only if they support the party line), is the chief reason why our benevolent government is suddenly so concerned with promoting the benefits of food irradiation. It wants that weapons-grade plutonium to fuel its plans for Star Wars and the other nuclear nightmares currently prevailing at the Pentagon. Will the American public allow itself to be hoodwinked once again? It is too early to say. On the plus side, at this writing the FDA will be requiring food treated with radiation to carry a symbol to that effect (though processed food containing irradiated ingredients will not!). The message is clear: Don't buy any food that has been irradiated. (The state of Maine has recently banned food irradiation.)

The question may arise in your mind, as it certainly has in mine, How did these gruesome situations develop? And how can they be promoted, camouflaged as reason? Given the known history of every aspect of nuclear energy and the effects of long- and short-term radiation on living organisms, it seems inconceivable that sane human beings should still be looking for legitimate uses for this grotesque technology. The social historian Lewis Mumford summed up the situation accurately and succinctly:

> Madmen govern our affairs in the name of order and security. The chief madmen claim the titles of general, admiral, senator, scientist, administrator, secretary of state, even president. And the most fatal symptom of their madness is this: they have been carrying through a series of acts which will eventually lead to the destruction of humankind, under the solemn conviction that they are normal, responsible people—living sane lives and working for reasonable ends. Why do we let these madmen go on with their game without raising our voices? Why do we keep our glassy calm in the face of this danger?
>
> There is a reason. We view the madness of our leaders as if it expressed a traditional wisdom, a common sense.

How to Fight the Conspiracy Against Your Health

It seems impossible to argue the fact: The least responsible people are entrusted with making the most momentous decisions. It is self-evident that the world is in a pickle, and it will almost certainly get worse before it gets better. Nevertheless, the present plight of our society should be viewed as the darkness before the dawn. Despite the conscious or unconscious opposition of government and industry, individuals everywhere are beginning to recognize where their own interests lie. Voices of sanity are beginning to make themselves heard. The natural health movement represents such a collective sane voice. In a way, the situation is better now than it was forty years ago when a voice such as my own was almost singularly crying out in the wilderness.

If we all take individual measures to stay healthy in our poisoned world, the future may yet be bright. The great social questions confronting humanity at the moment cannot be solved by sick people who have not solved their own personal problems. It's my conviction that individual health is absolutely crucial to the future health of our own society and the world at large. It stands to reason that if you are healthy yourself, you deal with your own personal world in a much more efficient and satisfactory way than if you are sick. A million healthy people or a billion healthy people will create a very different tomorrow from that created by a billion sick people.

The bottom line is that it's up to you, personally, individually. It is what I've been counseling my own patients for decades, and it works. Start now. Start with yourself. Start putting the right foods into your body and in the right combinations. Exercise, brush. And by healing yourself, you will be taking the first crucial step toward healing a sick society.

CHAPTER 11

The First Day of the Rest of Your Life

August 14th, 1972

Dear Doctor Soltanoff:

In early July when I painfully hobbled into your office supported by my wife and leaning heavily on a walking stick, I was convinced that I was destined for a wheel-chair for the rest of my life. While I WAS impresssed when you took the time to sit down with me— AND my wife—review the various foods I consumed, and the various ailments I suffered from, then analyzed my trouble and the cause of it, I must confess I was apprehensive when you assured me that if I cooperated fully, you could help me with my Arthritis etc.

You advised me that you could not cure me over-night, but I realized my Arthritis had not struck me over-night; it had developed over three agonizing years to the point where I was uncomfortable in any position and suffered continually night and day. Walking with support for even a few yards made me sweat with pain.

Doctor Soltanoff, while I still have twinges occasionally, my legs are getting stronger every day and on Sat., August 12th, after conducting a Wedding Ceremony in our Glenford Church, I attended the Reception, and—praise the Lord—for the first time in years, I ACTUALLY DANCED!

My friend, I don't have the words to adequately express my gratitude for all you have done for me, nor can I fully express my admiration of your God-given healing ability. I know you still want to work on me but I feel so wonderfully well I just HAD to write and say a warm and sincere "thank you!"

I would add, that by following your instructions concerning the types of food I consume, I have lost nine pounds, feel wonderfully healthy and have NOT felt any pangs of hunger.

Sincerely yours,

Reverend J. Filson Reid

I have this letter hanging on the wall of my office for all my new patients to see. I keep it there (and include it here) not to sing my own praises but to give my patients courage, because in order for your body to really heal itself, it takes time and hard work. Just as Reverend Reid's arthritis did not start overnight, it could not be cured overnight. But it *will* happen. Let's look at what happens to your body when you begin biochemical reprogramming.

After you start the natural healing program, you will at first find yourself making gratifying progress. But then you may suffer an apparent relapse. You may find your energy level suddenly depleted. There is often a feeling of letdown, lethargy, perhaps even depression and overall "blah." This is normal and almost unavoidable if a powerful stimulant (coffee, tea, chocolate, cocoa) is suddenly dropped from your diet. When a stimulant is suddenly withdrawn from the body, two things happen. First, the heart slows down slightly. It's only a resting phase, but it registers in the mind as decreased energy. Second, the body—freed from its daily dose of poison—immediately works to get rid of the accumulated wastes. Flushed from the tissues and transported through the bloodstream, these irritants may register in your consciousness as headache, for example. When we replace lower-quality foods with high-quality foods, the same process occurs, although to a lesser extent. This is because foods laced with spices, salt, and additives tend to be immediately stimulating to the body. Animal foods—meat, fowl, fish, eggs—provide a quicker hit than nuts, vegetables, and so on. The body reacts to them in the same way as other stimulants.

The Crucial Phase

Your body will now direct its energy toward detoxification. You will register this as fatigue. Don't worry. Don't give in and pick up where you left off! You are entering the crucial phase.

Increased energy is being used for internal rebuilding, so less energy is available for muscular work. How long the let-down lasts depends of course on how toxic you are. Some people will experience only a brief and mild let-down phase. For others, it will come and go over a long period of gradual improvement. Still others will have a prolonged let-down (three days to a week; more than a week is rare) before improvement takes hold and continues steadily.

The body's reasoning goes something like this: *Look at all this fine food coming in! Now we have a chance to clean up and rebuild. Let's get this excess bile out of the liver and gallbladder and send it to the intestines for elimination. Let's get this sludge moving out of the arteries, veins, and capillaries. These arthritic deposits in the joints need cleaning up. Let's get these irritating food preservatives, aspirins, sleeping pills, and drugs out of the way, along with these other masses of fat that have made life so burdensome for us for so long. Let's keep going until the job is done.*

To give in now, to go back to bad habits, would abort this all-important healing process. (NOTE: Caution is essential, however, if you are elderly or have been taking heavy medication and react strongly to the program. Ease off several days. Then try again in a modified manner.) To neglect and abuse your body is to set yourself up for serious diseases in the future. Look, if you were in perfect health, if you were bubbling with energy sixteen hours a day, if you were radiantly happy, I suspect you would not have picked up this book. But I don't think I'm being presumptuous to think that there is probably something wrong with your health, your energy level, or your emotional state.

Overtiredness, pain, nausea, indigestion, fever, colds—all these are the body's warning signs. If you understand these early symptoms and make the decision to take care of your body by cleaning out the poisons instead of bottling them up with a pill, no serious degenerative diseases will develop.

Looking in Vain for Instant Relief

Instant relief applies only to superficial, instant pain. Putting aloe on a mosquito bite is legitimate instant relief. Taking Rolaids or Tums for recurrent indigestion is not instant relief. Taking drugs or painkillers only injures the body further. So have faith! Wait out the let-down phase! Take the time to get the extra sleep and rest your body requires. After this period is over, the body's increased strength will far exceed the preprogram strength.

When to Start

The best time to start is now. Nevertheless, there are, as it were, good and better nows. Because of the energy required for detoxi-fication, you should try to initiate the program at a time when social and work obligations are at a minimum so that you can get the extra rest your body will need. Most of my patients find it easier to start on the program in the late spring or summer when the local markets are bursting with home-grown wholesome produce. This doesn't mean that you shouldn't start in the winter, just that it will take more initiative. It may be a good time to ease into the program by cutting the rubbish out of your diet. Give up the coffee. Start some sort of exercise program. Start skin brushing.

How to Start

This may sound self-evident. *What does he mean, "How to start"? You just start!* Believe me, it's not that easy. A habit is by definition hard to break. Every habit has a mind of its own, often a strong mind. Biochemical Reprogramming involves breaking bad habits. As if that weren't enough of an obstacle, there is often the most amazing opposition from family and friends. They will press drinks into your hand, ply you with coffee and cigarettes, and tell you they love you. They will call me an oddball, a quack, a charlatan, or worse and try to talk you out of following the program and, again, they will tell you they love you. I'm constantly amazed at the negativity that confronts patients who want to heal themselves. By now, as you know, Biochemical Reprogramming is self-healing. I don't heal my patients; they heal themselves. By way of illustrating both these points, let me tell you briefly the story of Alison A. Here are her own words:

> I might have gone blind in a matter of years. I had glaucoma, a gradual process, and the doctors couldn't seem to do anything to reduce the pressure in the eye. They gave me about six different medications to reduce the pressure and none of it seemed to work. I was at my wits end because they were tanking me up on about half a dozen different kinds of eye drops at once round the clock. I was feeling dizzy and nauseated, and I started to throw up a lot. It was as if I was seasick all the time.

Alison is a brilliant landscape painter. She came to me through other artists I treated in New York, and she was at her wits' end. Going blind is about the most traumatic event that can happen in anyone's life, but to an artist it is totally catastrophic, and there was no doubt that Alison was going blind. There was nothing wrong with the medical diagnosis. Alison had glaucoma alright, plus deterioration of the retina. What was wrong was the medication. Eye drops may relieve the pain, but do nothing for the condition. It's like wearing hip boots when the john is clogged. As is so often the case, her eye problem was a manifestation of deeper seated and chronic bodily imbalance. She went totally on the program, with great discipline, but at the same time was terrified of giving up her visits to the ophthalmologist, and in fact, I encouraged her to keep going. Initially, as I am stressing in this chapter, the condition actually got worse. The pressure in her eye increased (due to the release of toxic waste). Alison was a classic worst case scenario. Not only did the increased pressure continue for several months before leveling off, but once the healing process was initiated, there were a number of minor relapses over the course of a year. Now glaucoma is considered irreversible. The pressure is not supposed to go down. But that miraculous day arrived—after the pressure had increased and then leveled off—when her ophthalmologist pronounced a decrease in the pressure. The healing process had begun and after about a year on the program, the healing momentum increased almost exponentially. It's five years now, and Alison's glaucoma is vastly improved and she takes no medication.

But the point I started to make is that, frightening as this disease was in its own right, Alison also had to put up with constant flack at home. Her father, a powerful and wealthy businessman, tried every trick he knew to stop her from following the program, even though the doctors considered glaucoma an irreversible disease. And this is what I always consider amazing! After all, I was not stopping her from seeing her doctors, I wasn't telling her to stop the medication; I wasn't giving her any new or untried medications of my own. All I was doing was taking the poison out of her life and advising her to exercise and skin brush. Surely, at the very worst, I could not be doing any harm. But to Alison's father I was a quack, and it wasn't until his daughter started showing unmistakeable signs of recovery that he let up with the negativity. My advice therefore is that when you start Biochemical Reprogramming, be careful whom you tell—particularly when, like most everyone else, you go through that letdown period. Afterward—when you find yourself jumping out of bed wide awake at seven in the morning, working through the day with unflagging energy, never coming down with colds when everyone else around you is—that is the time to start talking about it.

There are three steps to getting into a swimming pool. First you make sure there's water in the pool. Then you test the water (optional). Finally you get into the water. But there are two equally right ways to get into the water. The first is to dive in headfirst. This may be a shock, but you're swimming in a split second. The other way is to ease into the pool gradually. Both approaches work with Biochemical Reprogramming. If you dive in off the deep end, headfirst, expect the shock and that bracing feeling that follows. If you ease in, it will take you longer to get in the swim, but you will be swimming no less effectively than the person who went in headfirst.

If the water looks too cold, try the gradual approach. Start with any element or aspect of the program, and see what it does. Begin by giving up your morning coffee and croissant or whatever it may be. Give it a couple of weeks and see if you notice the difference.

Brush when you get up. If you're not exercising, start. Do *some-thing*. My experience with thousands of patients has been that as long as they participated in just one aspect of the program, invariably (and I say that without any reservations whatsoever) they would get results, and these results would gradually convince them (even with a thousand little chocolate devils whispering in their ear) to partic-ipate in the rest. If you do nothing, obviously, nothing I can say or do is going to help you back to health. But if you do something, I can guarantee you: you will know the difference and you will know it soon. Others will know it, too.

The story of my patient, Maureen H., a politician and cabinet member of an English-speaking country, is, I think, a good illus-tration of many of the points about starting and staying on the program:

> I had been searching for a solution to my persistent health problems for several years when a back problem resulting from a fall led me to the doorstep of Dr. Jack Soltanoff. I had never been to a chiropractor and had never imagined ever going to one. As a trained nurse, I was used to the more traditional medical treatment. Dr. Soltanoff found a very serious back injury during his routine examination. The injury from a bad bicycle accident had been unde-tected for forty years and had almost reached the point where it would be very difficult if not impossible to cor-rect. I could now understand why I felt so terrible. Not only was my back injured, but as a result of the injury, my entire system was functioning well below average. I was not digesting or absorbing my food. The blood supply to all my organs was reduced and my nervous system was operating under a serious strain.
>
> I started on the long slow climb back. It had taken me, as it takes most of us, many years to reach the poor condition of health which I was in, and not enjoying. Dr. Soltanoff told me it would take time and discipline to get my health back. He said the first stage of improvement would be quite dramatic, and it was, and the second stage of improvement would be slow, and it was. We all want

to find an instant cure for all our ills, but there are no magic pills or cures that take the place of good eating and a healthy lifestyle.

I changed my lifestyle overnight.

Two chiropractic treatments a day began to correct the advancing curvature of the spine. I began a cleansing diet supplemented by vitamins. NO COFFEE, NO LIQUOR, NO SMOKING. (I was already a non-smoker.) Exercises for my back—swimming, walking, skipping, bicycle riding—all activities I loved, but had forgotten, also helped. I began to improve immediately.

At first I dropped below my natural weight from 128 lbs. to 118 lbs. I was too thin, and my friends and family were concerned about me. However, Dr. Soltanoff assured me that I was only losing poor quality tissue and I would replace it with stronger, healthier tissue. That is exactly what happened. I returned to my normal weight, but I dropped a complete dress size from size 10 to size 8.

I felt better and looked better. My skin improved and became clearer. I had more energy, and I also found, much to my surprise, that I could even think more clearly.

This is not a diet, it is a way of eating, a lifestyle. It suits my body's metabolism and it agrees with my attitudes and beliefs about health.

Health Returns in Cycles

Good health is pretty obvious. You know when you're feeling healthy and when you're not. Nevertheless, with Biochemical Reprogramming there are ups and downs, the process is gradual, and it's not always easy to determine objectively how you're doing. That is to say, how you feel on any given day is not necessarily a true reflection of your condition. But one of the nice little bonuses of Biochemical Reprogramming is the quick, painless, effortless, and almost free test described in Chapter 2. The pH test provides you with an objective assessment. You may not feel particularly radiant, but if your pH is steadily becoming more alkaline, you may be quite certain that your radiant days are not far off. The important thing to remember is the cyclical nature of healing. You're going to have

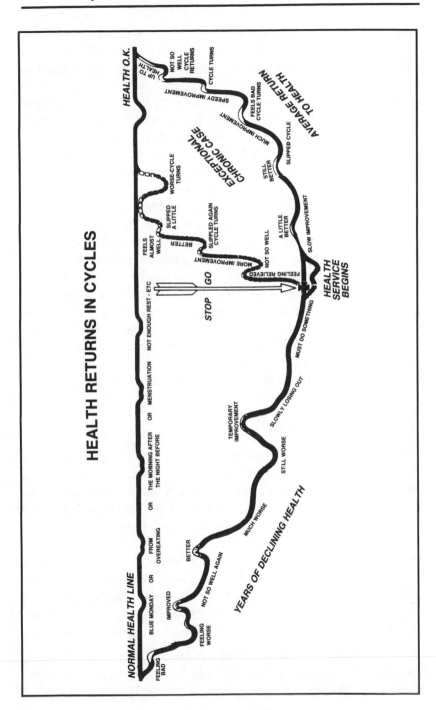

HEALTH RETURNS IN CYCLES

periods of relapse, usually brief, even if you haven't lapsed back into coffee or alcohol or whatever may have been your favorite bad habit. The chart on page 251 is a very rough visual approximation of the process. I say rough because the Ideal Health line should not really be horizontal. No matter how glowing your health at ninety, you will not be physically the person you were at twenty, though with a bit of luck you should be wiser. The Years of Declining Health line does not really reflect the specifics of an individual case or even an average case, but the general idea is accurate enough to illustrate the point. It is the Average Return to Health that is the most interesting to us. As you see, the general upward movement is gradual at first and then turns steep as the healing process accelerates. But throughout there are those periods of relapse. Again, this is an approximation. People with very long term chronic ailments cannot *all* expect a return to "ideal" health. The line showing the exceptional chronic case is the carrot on the stick. Every once in a while, perhaps a case in a hundred, somebody responds in the manner illustrated here. In these cases, recovery is almost miraculous. It happens. It could happen to you. The odds are considerably better than the lottery, and there's more at stake. But in this case, if you don't win, it doesn't mean that you lose. You win just the same, but slower.

Health as a Way of Life

Health is the result of living in accordance with the natural laws that govern our being. Most sickness' is a result of transgressing those laws. If you want to enjoy excellent health, you must make it a habit. The day-to-day actions that make for health and efficiency must become routine: eating, exercising, and caring for your body. No "get healthy quick" schemes, pills, operations, or hormone treatments ever take the place of small healthful acts repeated over and over again until they become the easiest and most natural way of living. If you practice healthful habits daily until they become a part of you, you will be rewarded by health you never dreamed possible. Start to build health by adopting the natural healing plan:

1. Eat more alkaline foods. There are two kinds of food, alkaline-forming and acid-forming. Alkaline-forming foods are fundamentally beneficial. Overalkalinity is no better than overacidity,

but it is very rare. Overacidity is the common condition of virtually everyone in twentieth-century America. Aim for a diet that is made up of 60 to 70 percent alkaline-forming foods. (See the acid/alkaline chart, pages 23–24.)

2. Combine your food properly. Foods must be eaten in the right combination to assimilate them effectively and get full benefit from them. Even good food will not guarantee you good health in wrong combinations. The glands feed upon body secretions and for health require living mineral and alkaline elements. The rule of thumb is fruit for breakfast; fruit *or* vegetables for lunch, with occasional dairy products; vegetables, especially salads, for dinner. Animal protein should only be eaten sparingly. Don't overdo cereals and grains.

3. Chew thoroughly.

4. Eat only when hungry.

5. Exercise. You can't get full benefit from your food—even when it is the best food rightly combined—without exercise of some sort. Make exercise an integral part of your life, not an afterthought.

6. Dry brush every morning. This feels so good, it should require little further encouragement. It should be something you do automatically every morning, like brushing your teeth.

7. Get plenty of rest. Staying up till all hours may make you feel heroic, but like much heroism, it's stupid. Rest when you're tired. Try to fit a siesta into your day.

8. Make fresh air a part of your life. Don't take no for an answer. Air is a food and it is as essential to health to breathe fresh air as it is to eat good food. When I had my practice in New York, I found that patients who should have been responding to the program quicker were responding much too slowly. It took me some time to determine that what was missing from their lives was fresh air. The lungs extract nutrients from the air and will also absorb poisons if the air is poisoned. Lung cancer from cigarettes is the most dramatic worst-case result of breathing poisoned air. But people who live in cities are condemned to breathing more or less poisoned air twenty-four hours a day. There is little or no respite. Fortunately, most people do not have to be coerced into leaving the city for a couple of days. If you are a city dweller, make an effort to get away for country or seaside weekends on a regular basis. Your health will improve dramatically.

9. Get ten or fifteen minutes of sunshine a day. It's now generally known that overexposure brings on skin cancers in extreme cases, and it ages skin in all cases. But if you don't get some sun, it will subtly but inevitably affect your health. Vitamin D from the sun helps the body absorb calcium, and getting sun on you helps Vitamin A utilization. You can sunbathe in colder weather than you think. Bundle up and let the sun get at you.

10. Don't become a fanatic. Moderation is as important as willpower. You won't be able to sustain your pace, and you'll give up if you go too crazy. Besides, fanatics bore everyone except themselves. What you are aiming for is a lifestyle that makes you happy as well as healthy, and if you are not happy, it is unlikely that you will be really healthy. Remember, you have two "eat what you want" days in the Biochemical Reprogramming system.

11. Enjoy them!

Follow these eleven rules and you will be on the road to health; to physical, mental, and emotional well-being. No one in his or her right mind could ask for more. And remember, it is not just the food you eat that determines that crucial alkaline balance. Rest and sleep are alkalizers. Exercise, fresh air, pleasure, laughter, conversation, enjoyment, love . . . all are alkalizers. Health to you!

Questions and Answers

Over the years I've been jotting down questions my patients ask before or after I give them a program to follow. I'm sure some of these questions have occurred to you as you've read this book.

Q. *I continually crave bread [after a considerable time of following the program]. Doesn't this mean that my body needs it?*

A. No. Don't trust your appetite. Some people never lose their craving for bread. It's a learned response. Your body doesn't need it, and gluten in large quantities builds up in your small intestine. This is how you abuse your body. Most of us have been brought up eating a lot of bread, and there is something about the smell of fresh-baked bread that tricks us into craving it. It's a curious thing, but even after patients have lost the craving for coffee, sweets, and other dietary vices, they go on craving bread. Resist it. Eat bread sparingly and try to toast it. Toasting breaks down complex starches into simpler starches for easier digestion. Better yet, get yourself into the habit of eating rye or rice crackers or rice cakes.

Q. *Tell me quickly about food combinations.*

A. Vegetables and fruits are golden foods with the lowest stress on the body. They should never be eaten together. Animal foods should be used in moderation. Don't eat proteins and starches together. Don't combine sweets with any other foods. When your sweet tooth acts up, try a piece of fruit instead of chocolate.

Q. *If I don't drink milk or take calcium tablets, how will I ever get enough calcium?*

A. You can get calcium from raw or lightly steamed corn, whole sesame seeds, dates, oatmeal, broccoli, most raw nuts (especially almonds), millet, molasses, kelp, dulse, and all green leafy vegetables.

Q. *When I switched to the foods you recommended, at first I felt great. But then I felt a letdown. Why is that?*

A. When you switch to superior foods and suddenly stop using stimulants such as coffee, tea, and chocolate, headaches are common. This is due to the elimination by the body of many toxins such as theobromine and caffeine. Animal foods such as meat, fowl, and fish are more stimulating than vegetable proteins, and therefore the lessening of animal foods produces a slower heartbeat than usual. Your body starts to throw off waste. You may get diarrhea, violent headaches, nausea, aches, and creaks. You say to yourself, "What has gone wrong?" but this is a good sign. (NOTE: If you get diarrhea, drink plenty of water.) This initial let-down, marked by a decrease in energy, lasts anywhere from three days to a week or even longer and is then followed by an increase of strength and energy. Tiredness and indigestion are warnings to the body, which is responding to years of neglect and abuse. (See chapters 2 and 11 for more details.)

Q. *Will I lose weight on your program?*

A. Weight will be lost in the initial stages while the body is cleaning out waste matter and burning up and eliminating superfluous adipose tissue. A rock-bottom weight is reached, and then new healthy tissues are built in all over again, thereby increasing the body's weight again. The original weight will never be regained fully if too much superfluous tissue had been carried in the first place.

Healthy tissue is the aim of nature. The weight reached under treatment will be right for the patient; however, it may vary from the "normal" rate based on height and age.

Q. *Your program sounds like such a slow, gradual process. Isn't there something I can do to feel better fast?*

A. The great majority of the American public is looking for fast, fast relief, but it's not the answer. However, if you're prepared to match your motivation with discipline, go on the Supreme Diet and stick to it to the letter. Brush and exercise also, and you'll feel better a lot faster than if you ease into the program. On the other hand, your condition is the result of many years of bad habits. Even before you felt sick your body was rebelling. Accept the fact that the healing process has got to take a certain amount of time.

Q. *Must I give up everything I love?*

A. The whole point of this program is that it is not intended as a restriction. It is designed to allow you to integrate it into whatever your lifestyle may be. I don't want a patient to feel as if I'm putting him or her in a pair of handcuffs or a strait jacket. It's very important to be happy. True, you have to cure yourself of bad nutritional habits practiced over a lifetime. I can't do that for you. But once you're over the hump, most of your cravings will disappear. It will no longer be a burden, and the two "eat what you want" days are there to allow you to indulge old habits in a way that is both systematic and harmless.

Q. *Why is a "more" vegetarian diet so good?*

A. A "more" vegetarian diet not only improves your health, it reduces your food bill. Besides, leaning more toward a vegetarian diet provides other more easily digested and assimilated nutritional constituents at a much more reasonable price. Of course, just avoiding meat doesn't mean you're eating healthfully. You must eat the right food in the right combinations. (See chapter 5 for more on diets.)

Q. *How can I believe that meat, chicken, eggs, and fish are non-essential?*

A. Many of us do not credit vegetables enough with their important place as basic body-building and protective foods. Habit (not health awareness) makes most people add a few small portions of wilted salad or some overcooked vegetables to their meals. A greater appreciation of raw or lightly steamed vegetables would do much in upgrading one's resistance and health. Most Americans overeat the various animal and meat products at mealtimes, making vegetables minor and unimportant items of food. It should be the other way around. Animal and meat products should be minimized, and vegetables should be stressed: the familiar lettuce, escarole, dandelion greens, celery, carrot, cabbage, cucumber, okra, parsley, sprouted seeds or beans, beets, Brussels sprouts, spinach, watercress, and all the rest. (See chapter 9.)

Q. *You don't say anything about drinking eight glasses of water a day. Isn't this essential?*

A. I disagree with the medical establishment, which recommends drinking eight to ten glasses of water a day. You only need that much if you're addicted to a high-fat, high-salt diet, to flush out the toxins. But this amount of water places a terrible burden on the kidneys. You're giving them no rest. You have an internal barometer—the hypothalamus—that signals you if you require water. If you're not thirsty, don't drink. On a proper diet practically all the water you need comes from fruits and vegetables. The only time I ever drink water (always distilled) is on a hot, humid day.

Q. *Don't you think the emotions bring on ill health?*

A. Of course they do. You can't divorce your body from your mind. Psychiatrists and psychologists often try to do this. If you're sick physically, how can you be healthy emotionally, and vice versa? You can't. An improvement in physical health is definitely going to affect you emotionally, and you'll be able to cope with situations you couldn't deal with if you were in poor physical health. You see, your body and your mind work together. There is now conclusive evidence that attitude affects healing. So if you're sick, it's absolutely essential that you enter into the healing process confident you are going to get well.

Q. *Would you approve of going to a medical doctor for any reason?*

A. I know I tend to come down hard on the medical profession. This is not to say there are not plenty of dedicated, sincere, and in recent years, even enlightened orthodox doctors. Much of my research material comes from their work. But apart from this minority, my conviction is that most of modern medicine is crisis medicine. It's what you do in an emergency. And there they shine. They're brilliant. If I had a heart attack and needed oxygen, I'd pray for a doctor nearby. If I got hit by a car and had a compound fractured leg and was bleeding to death, I'd want the paramedics on the scene. For emergencies, for certain kinds of surgeries—hernias or plastic surgery, for example—modern medicine is like nothing in history. But when it comes to the chronic diseases, the stress diseases that are the overwhelming majority of ailments, most standard medical procedure is useless. And more often than not, it's harmful. The medical establishment as a whole still refuses to look at illness as an unnatural state. It addresses the symptom instead of the cause. It knows practically nothing about prevention and often seems not to care. Only in the last few years have they begun to recognize the links between nutrition, exercise, and ill health. Even now they're barely aware of the dangers posed by pollution, chemicals, and so on. Despite the proven terrible side effects of so many of the drugs they routinely prescribe, they go on prescribing them.

So what is one supposed to do? Pat them on the back and say, "Good try"? As I said, there are definite signs of improvement in the medical profession, but in my opinion, the rate of improvement remains criminally slow. We're not talking about a difference in point of view. This isn't an academic dispute. It's not a question of whose theory is right or wrong. We're talking about the health of patients, and sometimes it's a question of life and death. My patients—almost without exception—represent failures of establishment medicine. Obstinacy on this level amounts to criminal neglect, in my opinion. If this sounds harsh, you should see my file of medical horror stories or listen to some of my patients.

Q. *Why are you opposed to most drugs and medicines?*

A. The main reason is that they don't get at the *cause* of the disease; they just suppress the symptoms. They interfere with, they block, the body's natural curative powers. Drugs often produce side effects worse than the condition they're meant to cure. I feel pretty much the same way about drugs as I feel about orthodox doctors. They are something you resort to in emergencies. Americans have been buffaloed into believing that miracle cures can be brought about by miracle drugs. In my opinion, overprescription of drugs and overuse of over-the-counter drugs are both major factors in the prevalence of chronic disease.

Q. *What about you, Dr. Jack, what do you eat?*

A. My staples are baked potatoes, salads, and millet. I don't eat breakfast, and for years I've not eaten lunch. As you get older, even when you get plenty of exercise, you can get along on much less food than in your younger days. For dinner most days I have a baked potato or baked yam and a big salad, or millet and a big salad, usually between five and seven o'clock. That gives me all the proteins, vitamins, and minerals I need in the right combinations. I'll have brown rice every once in a while, avocado, chick-peas, and I snack on fruit around nine or ten at night. I eat a lot of seasonal, local fruits and vegetables. Fresh raw corn in the summer instead of potatoes. I eat nuts and seeds, soaking them overnight because that makes them easier to digest. (It's a trade-off—you gain digestibility, give up crunchiness.) Maybe two or three times a year if I'm eating out on special occasions, I'll have animal protein. The truth is, I don't really enjoy it anymore. About once a week after a movie or the theater, I'll have a high-quality ice cream. Since I lost my wife I've been on my own, so I cook less and eat more simply than I did before. My diet may not get such high marks among gourmets, but it tastes fine to me and is certainly nutritionally ideal. It's perfect for anyone living alone, on the go, and determined to eat right.

Q. *I've heard alfalfa is good for arthritis. What about that?*

A. Most people with arthritis have a buildup of uric acid, which often interferes with the absorption of many minerals. Alfalfa roots grow deeply and absorb a great deal of minerals and vitality from the earth. One of the most alkaline foods, it actually *remineralizes* your body. Alfalfa tablets soak up uric acid almost like a blotter. Here's what I suggest:

The first week, take two alfalfa tablets after each meal and two at bedtime (eight tablets a day). After that, on an indefinite basis, take twelve tablets a day, three after each meal and three at bedtime. Alfalfa tablets are a food, not a medication, so you can eat up to twelve tablets a day without worrying about overdosing. (Alfalfa tablets should be kept under refrigeration.) I also tell my arthritic patients to cut out all grains except millet, (and in limited quantities, buckwheat groats and brown rice) and taper off animal and dairy products. I also recommend eating alfalfa sprouts daily.

Q. *What do you do for colds?*

A. A cold is not the great mystery it's made out to be. It's simply an accumulation of waste in the body. A cold is the body's way of doing housecleaning. The body is trying to unload through the lungs, nose, or sinuses. But people object, "How can that be? I've got a cold, and I've infected everyone in the house." But after a bit of detective work, I find out that "everyone in the house" is eating and drinking the same wrong things. So they get colds. I'm exposed to colds all the time and very rarely do I catch one.

Here's what I advise for a cold: At the first sign of a cold, take an enema with lukewarm water, hold it as long as you can, and then expel it and rest for five minutes. Repeat (two to four times usually) until nothing comes out except liquid.

Now squeeze a lemon into a cup of very hot, but not boiling, water. Sip it slowly. Repeat every three hours for the entire day. If you get unbearably hungry, cut up and eat a grapefruit two or three times during the day. But lemon juice alone is better if you can stick to it. You should wake up in the morning on the mend.

If the cold is firmly entrenched, take enemas the first day and follow the lemon juice/grapefruit regime for two more days.

Q. *I know you recommend a daily rest of thirty minutes to an hour. Wouldn't a slantboard be even better?*

A. Twenty minutes on a slantboard is equivalent to two hours of sleep. A slantboard is a six-foot padded board set up so that you are lying down with your feet eighteen inches higher than your head. If you lie on a slantboard, you reverse the pull of gravity and relieve the pressure of your internal organs against one another. *Warning*: If there's a suspicion of high blood pressure, heart problems, or cardiovascular disease, don't use a slantboard because you could burst a blood vessel.

Some of you may remember Gaylord Hauser, one of the pioneers of nutrition in the 1920s and 1930s. Hauser was a handsome, charismatic lecturer. His lectures were standing room only. At the beginning of the talk he'd say, "Ladies, the greatest beauty treatment in the world is"—he'd pause, and everyone would strain to hear—"a slantboard."

Q. *Is it ever too late to start your program?*

A. Again, it's a question of degree. The program won't get you leaping off your deathbed. But if you can walk into my office under your own steam, the chances are the program will help you. Let me tell you about my friend Isadore Katzowitz, whom I met socially in Florida when he was in his early fifties. He had a bad duodenal ulcer and was going downhill fast under strong and useless medication. Then he heard about the link between nutrition and disease and started reading up on it. He totally changed his eating habits, started exercising, and the ulcer disappeared. He's now in his mid-eighties. He plays tennis every day, and his stamina is almost unbelievable. I'm in very good shape for my age, but I can't keep pace with Isadore. Isadore keeps a stack of health books in the back of his car and passes them out to potential converts.

Q. *Do you know of a cure for AIDS (acquired immune deficiency syndrome)?*

A. Before we talk about a cure, let us talk about the cause. Medical science is spending a vast amount of time and money trying to isolate a virus or some other material cause. I'd rather look at what is making the immune system vulnerable in the first place. AIDS is not a disease in itself. It is a breakdown of the immune system, leaving the victim wide open to a host of diseases. Under ordinary circumstances, these diseases might not be lethal. With AIDS, the defenses are down, and the diseases become lethal.

What has done this to your immune system? Our whole society, our whole way of life, is designed to wreak havoc with it. Everyone's immune system is under constant attack. Most people eat a poor diet. Add to that sedentary living, stressful or uncreative jobs, broken and unhappy homes, overprescribed drugs and over-the-counter drugs, and the billions of contaminants, pollutants, additives, and chemicals in our air, earth, food, and water supply.

Let's look at the main groups affected by AIDS: homosexuals, Africans, Haitians, drug users, and blood recipients. If you look into the lifestyles of all these groups with AIDS, you'll find that all of them, for different reasons, are made up of people whose immune systems are under particularly heavy fire. (Blood recipients themselves are not necessarily under heavy fire, but certain groups of blood donors are.) I feel confident that sooner or later medical science is going to recognize these factors as the chief cause of AIDS, even though it can't isolate them and measure them or vaccinate against them. So the real approach to AIDS is to build up the immune system, especially of those people or groups that are the most vulnerable. Meanwhile, I'd like to say that I think the relationship between normal heterosexual sex and AIDS is blown way out of proportion. It's the state of your immune system that is the important thing, not your sexual habits or even your sexual preferences.

Q. *Do you consider eggs animal protein, and are they a healthful food?*

A. Eggs come from chickens, so they are an animal protein. Egg yolks, if they come from fertile, free-range, barnyard eggs, are definitely good for you in small quantities. They are alkaline-forming, very high in Vitamin A, and easily digestible when eaten with a green salad and a tomato. On the other hand, egg white is acid-forming and hard to digest. Eat fertile eggs—yolks only—but sparingly.

Q. *Have you any specific recommendations for constipation?*

A. Yes. In fact, constipation can be a major factor in many serious ailments: arthritis, liver, gallbladder, and kidney problems. Prunes work, but they are highly acidic. To relieve constipation, try instead beets, beet tops, cabbage, broccoli, or black mission figs, which are alkaline-forming. Powdered whey and molasses taken separately or together also work. On a temporary basis, drink a few glasses a day of distilled water. Most important, get off the concentrated foods—meat, milk and milk products, refined flours, and sugar— that brought on the constipation in the first place. Another big factor in constipation is inactivity—so start exercising.

Q. *Do multiple sclerosis patients respond to your program?*

A. Generally speaking, MS patients respond favorably, but some do not. MS is brought on by the erosion of the myelin sheath of the nervous sytem. Apparently, good nutrition can gradually help restore it to health. Recovery, however, may take a long time, depending upon the patient's age, the degree of the patient's commitment to a healthful diet, and the stage of the disease.

Q. *What can you do for PMS [premenstrual syndrome]?*

A. There are two factors usually involved in PMS, and it can involve one or the other, or both. First, there is often an unsuspected spinal problem. The lumbar spine may be displaced, not enough to actually hurt but enough so that it blocks nerve transmission to the ovaries and uterus. If this is the only cause, then chiropractors and osteopaths often get miraculous results with just a couple of treatments. The other factor is nutritional. The American diet makes everybody toxic (alcohol is a particularly significant factor in many PMS cases). And the toxins tend to sensitize the breasts and the reproductive tract in women, bringing on PMS. A change of diet and temporary vitamin and mineral supplements—magnesium, calcium, and selenium—usually works wonders, even on long-standing problems.

Q. *What do you know about chronic Epstein-Barr virus [CEBV]?*

A. Like many other practitioners, I'm not so sure it's a virus. I'm inclined to think that those who say it's a new name for an old disease are on the right track. CEBV has been described as endless mononucleosis with a touch of Alzheimer's. Doctors have found it difficult to diagnose and treat. According to my reading, the only really effective treatment so far has been nutritional and/or psychotherapeutic. Certainly the symptoms correspond to the symptoms of patients who have come to see me over the years; in the past my own evaluation would have been generalized toxemia. Again we are dealing with a failure of the immune system. And even orthodox medical circles recognize that a combination of bad diet, stress, and general pollution can depress the immune system. CEBV people tend to test out highly acidic, and the change of lifestyle and nutritional program has proven effective. CEBV, called the yuppie flu, seems to affect single people and/or people in high-stress jobs. I believe that just as malnutrition is the hidden factor in so many chronic ailments of the elderly, so here a different kind of malnutrition is the culprit in CEBV.

Q. *Sticking to your program seems to make it impossible to eat out. What about business lunches or a job that requires a lot of socializing?*

A. Unless you're really sick, my program includes two ''eat what you want'' days. If that's not enough for your schedule, a little ingenuity is the answer. There are always baked potatoes, salads, vegetables, fruit plates, and sometimes an acceptable soup. Even some fast-food restaurants have them. You can always bring your own herbal tea bag or ask for a cup of hot water and a lemon. Most restaurants will oblige. Initially that may sound restrictive, but I can guarantee you, once you're on the program awhile and you start to feel the benefits, most of your old restaurant habits will pretty much disappear. The major plus of following the program at restaurants is your energy level when you leave. You'll find that the after-lunch or after-dinner heaviness that you always considered a natural result of your meal is a thing of the past. It just doesn't happen when the digestive system is given a break from all that heavy food.

Q. *I'm confused about coconut. I hear it's a heavily saturated fat like butter or cream. But you recommend it highly.*

A. Remember, I'm talking about raw coconut, not coconut oil. It is true that coconut has a high saturated fat content, but it's a wonderful source of easily digested nonanimal protein. If it's taken in a shake with lecithin granules, the lecithin neutralizes the fat. When you eat it raw along with other fresh fruit, or a salad, the same thing happens. Its value as an appetite suppressant is generally overlooked by nutritionists, who frown upon it. Concentrated coconut oil, on the other hand, is no different from eating lard. Many processed foods use coconut oil because it's cheap. Don't eat processed foods that contain coconut oil.

Q. *How about cataracts? Surely they aren't brought on by bad diet.*

A. In most cases, people with cataracts tend to eat large quantities of dairy products. In my view, cataracts are a kind of arthritis of the eye. That film is excess calcium the body hasn't been able to eliminate. I don't say diet will cure cataracts, but they will respond to nutrition depending upon the seriousness of the condition and the seriousness of the patient in following the program. In the final analysis, a cataract is not an eye problem, it's a body problem.

Q. *Can I be assured of finding reliable products in health food stores?*

A. It's a question without a simple answer. Many health food stores are run by dedicated, conscientious people who make sure (insofar as they are able) to carry legitimate products and genuinely organic foods. At the same time, as soon as there is money to be made, rip-off artists appear as if by spontaneous generation. You have to judge for yourself, read the labels, and test your general impression of the way the place is run. Chances are you will never meet the chairman of the board of your local supermarket chain, and it will be impossible for you to judge his honesty, his values, or his ethics. But it's highly likely that you'll have some sort of personal relationship with the proprietor of your local health food store. Trust your judgment. Beyond that, there are highly reputable mail-order sources that I know you can depend upon, and there is now a movement devoted to organic greenhouse culture supplying genuinely organic produce in winter.

Q. *I'm worried about the way my parents eat. What can I do?*

A. Malnutrition is one of the chief unrecognized factors in diseases of the elderly. Let me tell you a story about Lou C., the father of one of my friends. This was a strapping guy in his seventies who was wasting away and wasting away fast. Contrary diagnosis called it lupus, then arthritis, then Alzheimer's. He was in three hospitals and the Westchester Medical Center. They put him on massive doses of painkillers and cortisone. They told him not to worry: Arthritis was common at his age and not life-threatening. Actually, he was deteriorating fast. By the time I got to see Lou, all his joints were fused, and the situation was hopeless. I could see that what was at issue was prolonged malnutrition. This not-so-old widower, formerly a great carouser and gourmet cook, had caught a severe cold and never fully recovered. His energy level was down to such an extent that he couldn't bother to cook for himself or go out for restaurant food. He put himself on a permanent diet of frozen dinners and other so-called convenience foods. Within eight months he was in the hospital. No one even suspected malnutrition. Yet it is just this that is behind the illnesses of a large percentage of our ailing senior citizens. Get your parents on a good nutrition program.

Q. *Your program contradicts a lot of the standard health practices I've been brought up with. Where's the evidence that your ideas are right and the others mistaken?*

A. My information comes from research. I've got a library with 6,000 volumes in it collected over the years. About 75 percent of those books relate to my practice in one way or another. Most of those books are written by scientists, many of them by practitioners like myself (who are writing as a result of personal experience), and some of those books are written by M.D.'s or other academically qualified sources who've also recognized the inadequacy of the standard view. So my evidence is not something I've dreamed up out of thin air but a kind of condensation of a lifetime of reading and practice. The practice is my clinical research.

Look, my patients usually come to me as a last resort, because they've tried all the orthodox conventional treatments and they haven't worked. They are sick in the first place because they've listened to a lot of propaganda and misinformation put out by vested interests: the dairy industry, the meat industry, food processors. When they get on my program, they usually get better. It's as simple as that. As far as I'm concerned, healthy patients are the only evidence that means anything when it comes to health.

Foods for Beauty

Natural beauty has little to do with perfect features. It is an indefinable magnetic quality made up of good health, clear skin, sparkling teeth and eyes, healthy hair, and above all, character and expression.

I am constantly amazed at women who assault their skin and hair with chemicals they wouldn't dream of drinking or eating. But as we know, the skin is an absorptive organ. Put poison on your skin, and it will soon find its way into the internal organs. Cosmetic companies may list ingredients on their labels, but they are not obliged to submit their formulas or safety data to the FDA. Of course, it would help if we knew exactly what went into those delicate-looking, sweet-scented cosmetic mixtures. It seems to me common sense that it would be best for your hair and skin to play it safe. Choose natural cosmetics made from herbs and plants that have withstood the test of time, that have been used for centuries, and that have beneficial as well as cosmetic qualities.

Among these truly natural ingredients you will find such appetizing substances as cucumber, honey, fruit juices, and vegetable oils. Herbs are popular ingredients, particularly rosemary, chamomile, and lavender. Essential oils, obtained by distilling flowers, are used to impart a delicate fragrance that stimulates circulation.

Don't be deceived by the vast crop of "natural" foods and cosmetics that are continually advertised in the media. All too often these are synthetic chemical products with an infinitesimal amount of herbal and natural ingredients added for camouflage to exploit today's "natural" health boom. Your best shopping area for natural cosmetics is a health food store.

As far as soap is concerned, castile soap is the mildest. It has an olive-oil base and is best for delicate or dry skin. Glycerine or transparent soap is good for average skin. Tar soaps are best for oily scalp and skin. Many of the imported soaps—Spanish, English, German—are totally or relatively free of additives. They are sometimes hard to find. Try health food shops or specialty shops. Never use anything but castile soap on babies. To my knowledge, the only commercially available soap that is scientifically mild is Dove.

The majority of cosmetics sold in health food stores ban synthetics from their formulas—but not all. A few cosmetic companies do add small amounts of preservatives to prolong the otherwise short life of their products.

Unfortunately, there are no hard-and-fast rules by which you can tell whether cosmetics are natural or not, but once you find one that suits you and that you are getting results with, you might find it worthwhile to write to the manufacturer for a list of ingredients. Their reply can reveal an interesting story, besides giving you confidence in the cosmetic you are using. For instance, it's nice to know that the creams and lotions you are using are made from herbs and plants freshly picked on the day the products were made. You will also find that most natural cosmetics companies operate on a small scale, even to the extent of producing many products by hand, which adds a nice personal touch to the big business of beauty.

Vegetable oils can be used in any cream or lotion and also added to any facial to combat dry skin. All of these oils have the ability to penetrate the outer skin slightly and therefore aid in the lifetime need to lubricate and soften the skin. The best oils in order of value to the skin are coconut, avocado, almond, extra virgin olive, vitamin E, safflower, corn germ, olive, sunflower, sesame, and soy.

Wheat germ and wheat germ oil are both soothing and healing to the skin. The oil is better on the skin, as it contains more of a concentration of vitamin E.

Zest is the peel of citrus fruits. Use orange rind for a mild face massage and complexion softener. Use grapefruit or lemon rind for soft hands and elbows.

Cucumber has an excellent effect on the skin because it tends to even out the acid/alkaline balance. Peeled cucumber may also be used to cool the skin and to ease sunburn. It can also be used as an astringent, in hand lotions, and as an added beneficial ingredient in facials.

Dandelion is exceptionally high in vitamin A. Eating the flowers and leaves raw in salads helps clear the complexion and cleanse the body, and is also a liver cleanser.

Eggs are excellent conditioners. A good hair conditioner consists of three egg yolks and a few drops each of glycerine, cider vinegar, and safflower oil (oil should be at room temperature). Add together and rub through hair a half hour before washing. For a dry-skin facial, beat one egg yolk together with a tablespoon each of honey and vegetable oil and five drops of cider vinegar. Apply to a clean face. Rinse with tepid water. Close pores with cold water or a mild astringent.

Fennel may be used as a facial steam to prevent wrinkles. Bring one pint of water to a boil in a pot, and pour it over two tablespoons of ground-up fennel seeds in another pot. Turn down the burner under the pot, and drape a towel over your head, shoulders, and the pot to direct the steam to your face. Be careful not to catch the towel on fire. Then close your pores with cool water or an astringent.

Grapefruit has an inner membrane that has skin-softening powers. This can help chapped hands, elbows, rough knees, and the backs of legs.

Honey acts as a moisturizer and skin softener and is a reliable healer for certain skin eruptions. Dissolve one cup of raw honey in enough boiling water to create a watery consistency. Add two cups of milk and set aside. Dissolve one-half cup of sea salt and two tablespoons of bicarbonate of soda in a cup of warm water. Combine both mixtures in a quart jar. Add the entire mixture to a lukewarm bath and soak in it.

Apples can be used to help a dry skin. Core, pare, and chop a medium-sized apple. Soften into a mash. Add one-half teaspoon of milk or cream and one tablespoon of honey. Wash your face or use a cleansing cream first, and then apply the mixture as a mask. Wash off after twenty minutes, then rinse with tepid water, closing the pores with cold water.

Avocado. To prepare an avocado face and neck mask, peel half an avocado, then mash with a fork. Add one teaspoon of runny honey and one teaspoon of heavy sweet cream. Beat together well. Thoroughly clean face and neck, then apply the avocado mixture liberally to these areas. Lie down, relax, and let it sink in for ten to fifteen minutes. Remove the mask with a face cloth dipped in warm water, and "rest" your skin by not using any makeup for at least two to three hours following the facial. If any mask is left over, use it on rough hands and feet. Many cosmetic firms use avocado oil in their skin-treatment products. They've known about its lush effects on the skin for a long time.

Lemons. To relieve dandruff, rub lemon juice into the scalp after shampooing. To brighten the hair, add the juice of one lemon to the final rinse water after shampooing. To soften and improve the quality of the skin, dilute one lemon in rose water. Lemon is also an astringent. Use it to cleanse and tighten skin.

Potato. A potato raw and peeled can be rubbed on the face or body to help clear up blemishes. For an excellent hand cream, mash two cooked medium potatoes, add a tablespoon of glycerine, several drops of rose water, and a tablespoon of safflower or almond oil. Blend these together into a thick paste and gently rub on your hands. Leave on for five minutes, then wash off with tepid water.

Brewer's yeast, helpful for normal, dry, or oily skin, is an aid for wrinkle prevention when used regularly on a long-term basis. Yeast facials are effective because they bring increased circulation to the face. Oil the skin lightly before applying the facial. Then dissolve one-half teaspoon of brewer's yeast in a small amount of water. Add one tablespoon each of honey and vegetable oil and one-fourth teaspoon of cider vinegar. Blend together. Do not apply more than once a week (yeast can irritate the skin of the neck—do not use on the neck.)

Sea Salt can be used to rub off dead skin cells. It is also an inexpensive mouthwash and tooth powder. For a mouthwash, add a tablespoon of salt to water. For a tooth powder and tooth cleaner, mix half salt and half bicarbonate of soda, moisten, and gently brush both teeth and gums with a moderately soft toothbrush.

Cider vinegar helps prevent flaky skin and excessive dryness and helps control dandruff. It makes an excellent hair rinse. When vinegar is used for the skin, water must be added to it in proportions of eight of water to one of vinegar. *Note*: Never use white vinegar, which contains a harmful chemical substance (acetic acid).

Tea. To reduce undereye puffiness, apply brewed eyebright tea on soaked cotton pads under eyes frequently.

Aloe. An aloe plant should be in everybody's home. The aloe has both medicinal and cosmetic properties. It can be used as an astringent. It will tighten and moisturize the skin. It takes the sting out of sunburn and mosquito bites. It also works wonders on burns. A liquid aloe gel can now be found in health food stores, pharmacies, and even supermarkets.

Mail Order

ALASKA
Briggs Way Company
Ugashik, Alaska via
King Salmon, AK 99613

Briggs Way natural Alaskan salmon canned in glass. Salmon is packed in glass containers because glass does not alter the fresh salmon flavor. To keep the salmon strictly fresh, it is iced within minutes and processed within hours. A gourmet's delight. 12.5 oz. jars $35 postpaid. Write for large quantities.

ARIZONA
Arjoy Acres
HCR Box 1410
Payson, AZ 85541
(602) 474-1224
Garlic, elephant garlic, shallots.

ARKANSAS
Country Bazaar
Rt. 2, Box 190
Berryville, AR 72616
(501) 423-3131
Honey bee pollen. Bee pollen, propolis and royal jelly in honey.

Mountain Ark Trading Company
120 South East Ave.
Fayetteville, AR 72701
(800) 643-8909
Vegetables, miso, seasonings, rice, pasta, fruit, spreads, oils, beans, soup. Certification varies; products labeled accordingly.

Organic Beef, Inc.
P.O. Box 642
Mena, AR 71953
(501) 387-7111
Organic beef has no added hormones, antibiotics, nitrites or other chemicals. Great for heart patients and allergy patients. Specialize in lean, low cholesterol beef. Shipped direct—frozen and packed in dry ice. Call or write. Evening calls welcome.

Ozark Cooperative Warehouse
401 Watson St.
Fayetteville, AR 72701
(501) 521-COOP
Refrigerated delivery of 1300 natural food products. Forty different Wisconsin cheeses, fruit juice, fruit juice sodas, snacks, organic grains, beans and produce. Free newsletter and pricelist.

Pine Ridge Farms
P.O. Box 98
Subiaco, AR 72865
(501) 934-4565
Organically grown chicken. Straight from an old-fashioned farm to you. One hundred percent chemical free. No additives, USDA inspected. Shipped direct—frozen and packed in dry ice.

Riverdell Gardens
Gordon & Susan Watkins
HGR 72, Box 34
Parthenon, AR 72666
(501) 446-5783
Organically grown strawberries and specialty vegetables.

Rock Crescent Ridge Farm
202 E. Church
Pocahontas, AR 72455-2899
(501) 892-9545
Vegetables, lambsquarter, Jerusalem artichokes.

Southern Brown Rice
P.O. Box 185
Weiner, AR 72479
(501) 684-2354
Organically grown brown rice. Excellent quality at fair prices. Hulled after you order to insure freshness. Short, medium, and long grain brown rice; basmati and wild rice available.

Ned & Pamela Whitlock
Star Rt. 1, Box 140
Osage, AR 72638
(501) 553-2550
Apples and pears. September-November.

CALIFORNIA
Lee Anderson's Covalda Date Co.
51-392 Hwy. 86
P.O. Box 908-N
Coachella, CA 92236
Dates, citrus, and nuts. 30 years organic. Retail and wholesale. Write for price list. Visit packing plants and Natural Food store.

Be Wise Ranch
Bill Brammar
9018 Artesian Rd.
San Diego, CA 92127
(619) 756-4851

Limes, lemons, avocados, oranges. A minimum order of 40 lbs. of citrus and 25 lbs. of avocados is required.

Ecology Sound Farms
42126 Road 168
Orosi, CA 93647
(209) 528-3816
Kiwi fruit, persimmons, Asian pears, plums, oranges, garlic, dried fruit.

G & J Farms
Gregory F. Gaffney
4218 W. Muscat
Fresno, CA 93706
(209) 268-2835
Apricots, peaches, assorted vegetables.

Giusto's Specialty Foods, Inc.
241 East Harris Ave. S.
San Francisco, CA 94080
(415) 873-6566
Breads, cakes, grains, spices, cereals, flour, oil, seeds, cookies, yeast.

Jaffe Bros. (NA)
Valley Center, CA 92082
Save on bulk buying. Flavorful, untreated dried fruits, nuts, seeds, grain, unrefined olive and sesame oils and other natural foods. 37 years shipping top quality organic foods. Free catalog.

Living Tree Centre
P.O. Box 797
Bolinas, CA 94924
Organically grown shelled almonds and almond butter. Send SASE for price list.

Joe Soghomonian
8624 S. Chestnut
Fresno, CA 93725
(209) 834-2772
Grapes and walnuts in season only, raisins year-round.

Sun Mountain Research Center
35751 Oak Springs Drive
Tollhouse, CA 93667
(209) 855-3710
Herbs, herb seeds.

Timber Crest Farms
4791 Dry Creek Rd.
Healdsburg, CA 95448
(707) 433-8251
A wide variety of dried fruits.

Treehouse Farms, Inc.
P.O. Box 168
Earlimart, CA 93219
(805) 849-2606
For the almond lover. Whole natural almonds for gift giving, cooking and snacks. Elegant Gold foil-lined gift boxes. 3 lbs. at $12.00
or 5 lbs. at $18.50. Economy bags 2½ lbs. at $9.95, 3½ lbs. at
$12.95, or 5½ lbs. at $17.95. Prices include shipping. Mastercard/
VISA accepted.

West Valley Produce Co.
726 South Mateo St.
Los Angeles, CA 90021
(213) 627-4131 or 629-1656
Fruits, vegetables. Certification varies; products labeled accordingly.

CONNECTICUT
Butterbrooke Farm
78 Barry Rd.
Oxford, CT 06483
(203) 888-2000
75 varieties of chemically untreated, open-pollinated, short maturity
seeds.

IDAHO
Brown Company
P.O. Box 69
Tetonia, ID 83452
(208) 456-2500 or 456-2629
Idaho potatoes, seed potatoes.

INDIANA
Rick Cole
Rt. 1, Box 238A
Carthage, IN 46115
Organically grown grains and stone ground flours, wheat, rye, kannch soybeans (edible).

Dutch Mill Cheese
R.R. 2
Cambridge City, IN 47372
Natural Amish-produced cheese. 17 varieties—no additives, preservatives, or chemicals.

IOWA
Country Store, Paul's Grains
2475-B 340th St.
Laurel, IA 50141
(515) 476-3373
Organically grown grains: wheat, rye, barley, buckwheat, corn, oats, edible soybeans, popcorn. Whole grain or stone-ground into flour and cereals. Also a 7-grain cereal mix and a 7-grain pancake-waffle mix. Organically-fed meats: beef, pork, lamb, chicken, turkey, and rabbit. Organic eggs, honey, sorghum; fresh fruits and vegetables in season. Write or call for free produce list. Tours available and free overnight camping. Can ship.

Frontier Cooperative Herbs
P.O. Box 299
Norway, IA 52318
(319) 227-7991
Herbs, spices.

Nature's Korner
Terry & Ellen Visser
Rt. 2, Box 302
Iowa Falls, IA 50126
(515) 648-9568
Bread from flour ground fresh from Arrowhead Hard Red Winter
wheat. Overnight delivery in Iowa UPS. Also fresh flours and or-
ganic health foods. Shopping list upon request.

Lavern Schweer
Route 3
Cedarfalls, IA 50613
(319) 266-9325
Natural Iowa beef. Organically raised and processed using no chem-
icals, antibiotics, or preservatives.

MAINE
Fiddler's Green Farm
R.R. 1, Box 656
Belfast, ME 04915
(207) 338-3568
Pancake, muffin, and spice cake mixes; breakfast gift pack including
pancake and muffin mixes, maple syrup, honey.

MARYLAND
Smile Herb Shop
4908 Berwyn Road
College Park, MD 20740
(301) 474-4288 or 474-8495
Fruits, vegetables. Certification varies; products labeled accordingly.

Tuscarora Valley Beef Farm
P.O. Box 15839
Chevy Chase, MD 20815
(301) 588-5220
Lamb, veal, beef, nitrite-free bacon, lower-fat chicken sausages.

American Spoon Foods
411 E. Lake St.
Petoskey, MI 49770
(616) 347-9030
Pancake and waffle mix made with organically grown Indian blue
corn, wild rice, wild berry preserves, wild pecans.

Country Life Natural Foods
109 Ave.
Pullman, MI 49450
(616) 236-5011
Beans, grains, seeds, nuts, raisins. Certification varies, products
labeled accordingly.

Eugene and Joan Saintz
2225 63rd St.
Fenville, MI 49408
(616) 561-2761
Fruits and vegetables in season.

Diamond K Enterprises
R.R. 1, Box 30
St. Charles, MN 55972
(507) 932-4308
Grains, flour, cereal, pancake mixes, nuts, dried fruit, sunflower
oil, honey, peanut butter, alfalfa seeds.

Living Farms
Box 50
Tracey, MN 56175
(800) 622-5235 (MN)
(800) 533-5320 (out-of-state)
Grains, beans, rice, wheat, sunflowers, sprouting seeds (alfalfa,
clover, radish).

Midheaven Farms Beef
Rt. 1, Box 404
Park Rapids, MN 56470
(218) 732-4866
Beef. Ships directly to consumers in the Minnesota area only.

MISSOURI
Joseph T. Miller
R.R. 3, Box 202
Dixon, MO 65459
Organically raised young chickens, strawberries and sweet potatoes
in season. Sweet potatoes shipped anywhere in U.S.A.

Sandhill Farm
Box 155
Rutledge, MO 63563
(816) 883-5543
Organically grown and processed sorghum syrup. 2½ lb. jar—on
the farm $4, postpaid $8: 1 gal. 12 lb.—on the farm $15, postpaid
$22. Inquire for larger quantity/wholesale prices. Assorted organic
fruits and vegetables in season.

MONTANA
May Organics
Box 175
Winston, MT 59647
(406) 443-7049
Organically grown meats, eggs, herbs, organic soil amendments,
fertilizers, and feeds.

NEW YORK
Chesnok Farm
R.D. #1, Marshland Road
Apalachin, NY 13732
(607) 748-3495
Shallots, garlic.

Deer Valley Farm
R.D. 1
Guilford, NY 13780
(607) 764-8556
Beef, pork, chicken, turkey, eggs, fruit, grains, herbs, juice, pasta,
oil, soup, spaghetti, spreads, seasonings, baked goods, confections,
nuts. Certification varies, products labeled accordingly.

Four Chimneys Farm Winery
R.D. 1
Hall Road
Himrod, NY 14842
(607) 243-7502
Wine, grape juice, wine vinegar, champagne. Alcohol cannot be shipped out of state.

Red Fox Farm
RD 1, Box 7
Sharon Springs, NY 13459
Pure maple syrup. Grade A, no chemicals or preservatives; made the old fashioned way; packed in attractive jugs. Postpaid to you $32 per gal.

NORTH CAROLINA
New Hope Homestead
Rt. 5
Murphy, NC 28906
Bee-gathered pollens from the fields and forests of the Chattachoee National Forest. Direct from beekeeper. 1–5 lb. $7.00 ppd., 5–10 lb. $6.50 ppd. Over 10 lb. $6.00 ppd.

OHIO
Mike Brodman
6409 E. Scipio Top Rd. 8
Republic, OH 44867
(419) 585-5852 evenings
Organically grown beef. Straight from the farm. No hormones, antibiotics, nitrites, or chemicals. Also organically grown grains—certified by the Ohio Ecological Food & Farming Association.

Millstream Market
1310-A E. Talmange Ave.
Akron, OH 44310
(216) 630-2776
Organic produce. Fruits, vegetables, nuts, grains, and food products. Send self-addressed stamped envelope for free price list. Ship by UPS.

Beekeeper
862 Northwood
Salem, OR 97301
Pollen 1 lb. $8.70, 2.5 lbs. $16.40, 5 lbs. $26.75, 10 lbs. $48.50.
Pure Royal Jelly—2 ozs. $18.50, 4 ozs. $32.50. Postpaid, insured.
Free catalog.

PENNSYLVANIA
Garden Spot Distributors
Rt. 1, Box 729A
New Holland, PA 17557
(800) 292-9631 (PA)
(800) 445-5100 (Eastern U.S.)
(717) 354-4936 (Western, U.S.)
Baked goods, cereal, dried fruit, nuts, seeds, grains, flour, beans, granola, tea, herbs.

Genesee Natural Foods
Rt. 449
Genesee, PA 16923-9414
(814) 228-3200 or 228-3205
Beans, seeds, flour, pasta, corn chips, rice cakes, raisins, apple juice, tea, nut butters (peanut, almond, hazelnut, cashew). Certification varies, products labeled accordingly.

Neshaminy Valley Natural Foods
421 Pike Road
Huntingdon Valley, PA 19006
(215) 364-8440
Grains, popcorn, beans, dried fruit, pasta, flour, cereals, seeds, nuts, miso, candy, pickles, tea, some macrobiotic products. Only a buying club of six households or more can order products.

Rising Sun Distributors
P.O. Box 627
Milesburg, PA 16853
(814) 355-9850
Beef, poultry, lamb, pork, fruits, vegetables, beans, seeds, grains.

Walnut Acres
Penns Creek, PA 17862
(717) 837-0601
Meat, fish, poultry, canned vegetables, cheese, grains, seeds, flour,
nuts, pasta, seasonings, dried fruit, juice, salad dressing, granola,
peanut butter.

TEXAS
O. D. Anderson
Box 1083
Rocksprings, TX 78880
Organic beef. Natural, lean, lighter cholesterol beef. Limited supply.

Arrowhead Mills
Box 2059
Hereford, TX 79045
(806) 364-0730
Whole natural foods. Many grown in the mineral-rich soils of Deaf
Smith County, Texas.

J. Francis Co.
Rt. 3, Box 54A
Atlanta, TX 75551
(214) 796-5364
Organic beef, pork, and poultry.

Hawkins Creek Farm
P.O. Box 6552
Longview, TX 75608
(214) 759-8820
Organically grown vegetables. Call or write for information.

Imperial Organic Farms
Rt. 2, Box 55
Winnsboro, TX 75494
(214) 365-2660
Garden fresh vegetables. Organically raised, no poisons. Availa-
bility in season: tomatoes, squash, asparagus, peppers, cucumbers,
blueberries.

Robert McIlroy III
Rt. 1, Box 113A
Lampasas, TX 76550
(512) 768-3396
Black Angus Morlean beef. Half or whole. Lab-tested lower in fat
and cholesterol. Ship in Texas only.

Nelson's
Box 507, Rt. 1
Paris, TX 75460
(214) 784-2665
Organic beef grazed on land fertilized naturally.

Wylie's Country Store
Route 5, Box 26
Hwy. 37 S.
Winnsboro, TX 75494
(214) 629-7111
Greenhouse-grown vegetables grown by organic methods on fertile
soil. Tomatoes, cucumbers, peppers, and herbs shipped anywhere
in the U.S. Good Health Breads baked with organic grains shipped
or at store. Request latest bulletin for details. Bread baked fresh
Sunday through Friday. Arrowhead Mills flour used in our country
bakery. Organic foods and organic garden center.

VERMONT
Hill and Dale Farms
West Hill—Daniel Davis Rd.
Putney, VT 05346
(802) 387-5817
Apples, apple vinegar. Certification pending.

The Wright Farm
Carroll and Darlene Wright
Enosburg Falls, VT 05450
Pure Vermont maple syrup. Chemical-free. Send for brochure.

VIRGINIA
Golden Acres Orchard
Rt. 2, Box 2450
Front Royal, VA 22630
Biologically grown apples, apple juice and apple cider vinegar.

Jordan River Farms
Huntly, VA 22640
(703) 636-9388
Grass-fed beef, free-range eggs, veal occasionally.

Magic Garden Produce
Rt. 3, Box 304
Edinburg, VA 22824
(703) 459-3376
Organically grown alfalfa, radish sprouts, apple juice, wheatgrass, watercress. Holiday turkeys and Rainbow Trout. Wholesale and retail.

White Oak Farms
Rt. 2, Box 2340
Front Royal, VA 22630
Organic potatoes. Biologically grown in the beautiful Shenandoah Valley of Virginia. Write for free price list and shipping dates.

WASHINGTON
Cascadian Farm
Star Route
Rockport, WA 98283
(206) 853-8175
Fruit conserves, dill pickles.

Homestead Organic Produce
Bilss Weiss
Rt. 1, 2002 Road 7 NW
Quincy, WA 98848
(509) 787-2248
Gourmet Sweet onions. A 10 lb. minimum order is required.

For personalized hygiene individual brushes should be used for each member of your family. You can save 10% on two and 20% when ordering three or more brushes.

THE BRUSH

This flexible vegetable fiber brush has been specially designed to the requirements of Dr. Soltanoff's unique dry brushing program. It fits neatly in your hand and follows the contours of the body insuring that you stimulate the sensitive meridians and acupuncture points. It's durable and washable.
$7 each

THE CHART

The attractive laminated chart (11″ x 17″) shows you the body's acupuncture points and diagrams of dry brushing techniques. You will find the chart a convenient, informative, and easy-to-follow display guide.
$5 each

Please send your order to:

Natural Health Brushes
PO Box #239
West Hurley, NY 12491

Specify item and quantity. Enclose check or money order payable to HEALTH AND BEAUTY BRUSH. Add $2 for postage and handling (immediate shipment). N.Y.S. residents add sales tax.